CONTENTS

INCREASED DRUG ABUSE: THE IMPACT ON THE NATION'S EMERGENCY ROOMS

HEARING

BEFORE THE

HUMAN RESOURCES AND INTERGOVERNMENTAL RELATIONS SUBCOMMITTEE

OF THE

COMMITTEE ON GOVERNMENT OPERATIONS HOUSE OF REPRESENTATIVES

ONE HUNDRED THIRD CONGRESS

FIRST SESSION

MAY 26, 1993

Printed for the use of the Committee on Government Operations

U.S. GOVERNMENT PRINTING OFFICE

85-837 CC WASHINGTON : 1995

For sale by the U.S. Government Printing Office
Superintendent of Documents, Congressional Sales Office, Washington, DC 20402
ISBN 0-16-046530-3

COMMITTEE ON GOVERNMENT OPERATIONS

JOHN CONYERS, JR., Michigan, *Chairman*

CARDISS COLLINS, Illinois
GLENN ENGLISH, Oklahoma
HENRY A. WAXMAN, California
MIKE SYNAR, Oklahoma
STEPHEN L. NEAL, North Carolina
TOM LANTOS, California
MAJOR R. OWENS, New York
EDOLPHUS TOWNS, New York
JOHN M. SPRATT, JR., South Carolina
GARY A. CONDIT, California
COLLIN C. PETERSON, Minnesota
KAREN L. THURMAN, Florida
BOBBY L. RUSH, Illinois
CAROLYN B. MALONEY, New York
THOMAS M. BARRETT, Wisconsin
DONALD M. PAYNE, New Jersey
FLOYD H. FLAKE, New York
JAMES A. HAYES, Louisiana
CRAIG A. WASHINGTON, Texas
BARBARA-ROSE COLLINS, Michigan
CORRINE BROWN, Florida
MARJORIE MARGOLIES-MEZVINSKY, Pennsylvania
LYNN C. WOOLSEY, California

WILLIAM F. CLINGER, JR., Pennsylvania
AL McCANDLESS, California
J. DENNIS HASTERT, Illinois
JON L. KYL, Arizona
CHRISTOPHER SHAYS, Connecticut
STEVEN SCHIFF, New Mexico
CHRISTOPHER COX, California
CRAIG THOMAS, Wyoming
ILEANA ROS-LEHTINEN, Florida
RONALD K. MACHTLEY, Rhode Island
DICK ZIMMER, New Jersey
WILLIAM H. ZELIFF, JR., New Hampshire
JOHN M. McHUGH, New York
STEPHEN HORN, California
DEBORAH PRYCE, Ohio
JOHN L. MICA, Florida
ROB PORTMAN, Ohio

BERNARD SANDERS, Vermont (Independent)

JULIAN EPSTEIN, *Staff Director*
MATTHEW R. FLETCHER, *Minority Staff Director*

HUMAN RESOURCES AND INTERGOVERNMENTAL RELATIONS SUBCOMMITTEE

EDOLPHUS TOWNS, New York, *Chairman*

HENRY A. WAXMAN, California
THOMAS M. BARRETT, Wisconsin
DONALD M. PAYNE, New Jersey
CRAIG A. WASHINGTON, Texas

STEVEN SCHIFF, New Mexico
STEPHEN HORN, California
JOHN L. MICA, Florida

BERNARD SANDERS, Vermont (Ind.)

EX OFFICIO

JOHN CONYERS, JR., Michigan
WILLIAM F. CLINGER, JR., Pennsylvania

RONALD A. STROMAN, *Staff Director*
CHERRI L. BRANSON, *Professional Staff Member*
BRENDA E. PILLORS, *Professional Staff Member*
KIMI WASHINGTON, *Clerk*
MARTHA B. MORGAN, *Minority Professional Staff*

INCREASED DRUG ABUSE: THE IMPACT ON THE NATION'S EMERGENCY ROOMS

WEDNESDAY, MAY 26, 1993

HOUSE OF REPRESENTATIVES,
HUMAN RESOURCES AND
INTERGOVERNMENTAL RELATIONS SUBCOMMITTEE
OF THE COMMITTEE ON GOVERNMENT OPERATIONS,
Washington, DC.

The subcommittee met, pursuant to notice, at 10 a.m., in room 2247, Rayburn House Office Building, Hon. Edolphus Towns (chairman of the subcommittee) presiding.

Present: Representatives Edolphus Towns, Donald M. Payne, Steven Schiff, Stephen Horn, and John L. Mica.

Also present: Ronald A. Stroman, staff director; Cherri L. Branson and Brenda E. Pillors, professional staff members; Kimi Washington, clerk; and Martha B. Morgan, minority professional staff, Committee on Government Operations.

OPENING STATEMENT OF CHAIRMAN TOWNS

Mr. TOWNS. The Committee on Government Operations, Human Resources and Intergovernmental Relations Subcommittee will convene.

The hearing is on "Increased Drug Abuse: The Impact on the Nation's Emergency Rooms."

I am delighted to welcome our distinguished witnesses this morning to discuss the growing crisis the Nation's emergency rooms face because of increased drug abuse.

On April 23, the Substance Abuse and Mental Health Services of the Department of Health and Human Services issued an annual report detailing the statistical evidence of hospital emergency room visits caused by the use of illegal drugs.

The report cited an alarming increase in the use of emergency rooms by heavy and long-term drug users. Of particular concern is the incredible increase in emergency room visits caused by the use of heroin.

In the late 1970's or early 1980's, there were reports that a purer, cheaper, and potentially more addictive form of cocaine was being sold on the American streets.

The alarm was sounded, but nobody listened. As a result, we have the epidemic of crack cocaine that is sweeping our streets, that is destroying lives, families, and communities day in and day out.

Today we sound the alarm again. Heroin is cheaper, purer, and in abundant supply. I hope we can learn from history. This report from Substance Abuse and Mental Health Services Administration is particularly important in pointing out the increases of heroin use. There are those who may draw the conclusion that the threat of widespread heroin use serves as an additional reason for long-term prevention and treatment efforts.

I do not disagree with them.

However, our Nation's emergency rooms are not the appropriate place for this kind of effort. The effect of this type of additional stress of substance abuse treatment on an overburdened emergency room system could prove disastrous to the 37 million individuals who lack health insurance and resort to the emergency rooms for nonemergency primary care. The emergency room must not become the center of substance abuse treatment for the poor.

I hope that today's hearing will point to the need not only for a serious program of substance abuse prevention and treatment but also to the need for available and accessible inner city prime health care facilities which are desperately needed throughout this Nation.

At this time, I would like to yield to the ranking member of the subcommittee, my good friend from Albuquerque, NM, Congressman Schiff.

[The opening statement of Mr. Towns follows:]

COMMITTEE ON GOVERNMENT OPERATIONS
HUMAN RESOURCES AND INTERGOVERNMENTAL RELATIONS SUBCOMMITTEE

HEARING ON THE

"INCREASED DRUG ABUSE:THE IMPACT ON THE NATION'S EMERGENCY ROOMS"

May 26, 1993

OPENING STATEMENT OF CHAIRMAN EDOLPHUS "ED" TOWNS

GOOD MORNING LADIES AND GENTLEMEN. IT IS A PLEASURE TO WELCOME OUR DISTINGUISHED WITNESSES HERE THIS MORNING TO DISCUSS THE GROWING CRISIS THE NATION'S EMERGENCY ROOMS FACE BECAUSE OF INCREASED DRUG ABUSE.

ON APRIL 23RD, THE SUBSTANCE ABUSE AND MENTAL HEALTH SERVICES ADMINISTRATION OF THE DEPARTMENT OF HEALTH AND HUMAN SERVICES ISSUED ITS ANNUAL REPORT

DETAILING THE STATISTICAL EVIDENCE OF HOSPITAL EMERGENCY ROOM VISITS CAUSED BY THE USE OF ILLEGAL DRUGS. THE REPORT CITED AN ALARMING INCREASE IN THE USE OF EMERGENCY ROOMS BY HEAVY AND LONG TERM DRUG USERS. OF PARTICULAR CONCERN, IS THE INCREDIBLE INCREASE IN EMERGENCY ROOM VISITS CAUSED BY THE USE OF HEROIN.

NOT SURPRISINGLY, THE MAJOR NORTHEASTERN CITIES WHICH HAVE TRADITIONALLY SERVED AS PORTS OF ENTRY FOR ILLICIT DRUG TRAFFIC , NEW YORK, PHILADELPHIA AND BALTIMORE HAVE EXPERIENCED THE HEAVIEST OVERALL INCREASES IN EMERGENCY ROOM VISITS ASSOCIATED WITH DRUG USE. THE PATTERN OF THESE STATISTICS ILLUSTRATES

THAT THE NATION'S EMERGENCY ROOMS SERVE AS A TRIAGE FOR A FAILED WAR ON DRUGS.

FOR THE LAST FEW YEARS, CONGRESSIONAL COMMITTEES, THE MEDIA AND HEALTH PROFESSIONALS HAVE WARNED THAT HEROIN HAS GAINED A NEW FOOTHOLD AMONG THE DRUG DEPENDENT SUBCULTURE. WHILE TELLING THE GOOD NEWS OF THE DECLINING USE OF COCAINE AND CRACK, THEY ALSO WARNED THAT THE NINETIES COULD PROVE TO BE A RETURN TO THE POPULAR DRUGS OF THE SIXTIES--HEROIN, LSD AND SPEED. I AM PARTICULARLY CONCERNED THE DRUG ENFORCEMENT ADMINISTRATION HAS FOUND AN INCREDIBLE INCREASE IN THE PURITY OF HEROIN CURRENTLY SOLD ON THE STREETS--UP FROM 5% PURITY IN THE SIXTIES TO ALMOST 50% PURITY TODAY. FINALLY BECAUSE OF THIS INFLUX OF ALMOST UNADULTERATED

HEROIN, THE PRICE IS EXTREMELY LOW. NOW IT SEEMS THAT AS THINKING PEOPLE, WE MUST TAKE NOTICE OF THIS. I REMEMBER IN THE LATE SEVENTIES AND EARLY EIGHTIES, THERE WERE REPORTS THAT A PURER, CHEAPER AND POTENTIALLY MORE ADDICTIVE FORM OF COCAINE WAS BEING SOLD ON AMERICAN STREETS. THE ALARM WAS SOUNDED BUT NOBODY LISTENED. AS A RESULT, WE HAVE THE EPIDEMIC OF CRACK COCAINE THAT IS DESTROYING LIVES, FAMILIES AND COMMUNITIES. TODAY, WE SOUND THE ALARM -HEROIN IS CHEAPER, PURER AND IN ABUNDANT SUPPLY. I HOPE WE CAN LEARN FROM HISTORY. THIS REPORT FROM SUBSTANCE ABUSE AND MENTAL HEALTH SERVICES ADMINISTRATION IS PARTICULARLY IMPORTANT IN POINTING OUT THE INCREASES OF HEROIN USE. THERE ARE SOME WHO MAY DRAW THE CONCLUSION THAT THE THREAT OF

WIDESPREAD HEROIN USE SERVES AS AN ADDITIONAL REASON FOR LONG-TERM PREVENTION AND TREATMENT EFFORTS.

I DO NOT DISAGREE WITH THEM. HOWEVER, OUR NATION'S EMERGENCY ROOMS ARE NOT THE APPROPRIATE PLACE FOR THIS KIND OF EFFORT. THE EFFECT OF THIS TYPE OF ADDITIONAL STRESS OF SUBSTANCE ABUSE TREATMENT ON AN OVERBURDENED EMERGENCY ROOM SYSTEM COULD PROVE DISASTROUS TO THE 37 MILLION INDIVIDUALS WHO LACK HEALTH INSURANCE AND RESORT TO EMERGENCY ROOMS FOR NON-EMERGENCY PRIMARY CARE. THE EMERGENCY ROOMS MUST NOT BECOME THE CENTER OF SUBSTANCE ABUSE TREATMENT FOR THE POOR. AND THEY MUST NOT CONTINUE AS THE CENTER OF PRIMARY AND NON-EMERGENCY CARE.

I HOPE THAT TODAY'S HEARING WILL POINT TO THE NEED NOT ONLY FOR A SERIOUS PROGRAM OF SUBSTANCE ABUSE PREVENTION AND TREATMENT BUT ALSO TO THE NEED FOR AVAILABLE AND ACCESSIBLE INNER CITY PRIMARY HEALTH CARE FACILITIES IN ANY OVERHAUL OF THE HEALTH CARE REFORM SYSTEM.

Mr. SCHIFF. Thank you, Mr. Chairman.

Once again, I want to express my appreciation for your willingness to work with our side to put together hearings on subjects that are important to all of our constituents, regardless of their political views.

And I think that you have selected a very important issue. Because in addition to the obvious health care problems to people that drug abuse represents, right now the administration is studying health care economic reform. And one of the problems that our system faces is the overuse of emergency rooms and the attendant per-hour cost that runs the system.

And you have correctly identified that drug overdose leads to a great amount of use of emergency rooms and that if we could find a way, as with any other health care problem, to address this issue before it becomes a crisis, then we can save the system a great deal of money, as well as, of course, saving the human costs involved.

And I thank you for scheduling this hearing, and I look forward to hearing the witnesses.

Mr. TOWNS. Thank you very much, Congressman Schiff.

Now, the person that is from the second fastest growing State in the Nation, Congressman Mica, from the State of Florida.

Mr. MICA. Thank you, Mr. Chairman. And I also want to commend you for convening this hearing on probably the most important social issue facing our Nation and that is drug abuse and its particular impact today on emergency rooms and hospital facilities throughout the country that are impacted by this disaster on our Nation.

But just by way of background, I had the good fortune of working in the U.S. Senate, the other body, for a number of years and oversaw a lot of the work over the drug panel chaired by Senator Paula Hawkins of Florida. And during the period I was there, from 1980 to 1985, we focused quite a bit on the enforcement side and through just about every type of resource we could against the problem of narcotics. I helped to author the current law which ties drug eradication into foreign aid of a country.

Some of those measures have worked. Some of them haven't. But we still see the impact on our emergency rooms and on our court dockets, in the destruction of the family, on the impact of crime. And so the problem is widespread.

I have looked at the issue. And just for your information, I will tell you and the other colleagues, people assembled, that I am really concerned that in drug education and prevention we have just scratched the surface to resolving the problem. And home, church, school, don't seem to provide the answers today.

I have identified television as one of the mediums that really has the biggest impact on our young people. And I intend to introduce, sometime this session, a bill to require that at least 5 percent of the commercial advertising on television be devoted to drug and substance abuse education and prevention because we control the airwaves that have such a tremendous impact. And maybe we can stop some of the impact on facilities such as hospitals, prisons, and social programs that are impacted.

So I just open with that little bit of background and information and again commend you for this important focus.

Mr. TOWNS. Thank you very much.

And at this time I would yield to Congressman Horn for any comment or opening statement he might have.

Mr. HORN. Thank you, Mr. Chairman.

I commend you and the ranking minority member for these hearings and your collaboration on it. Coming from California, obviously, we are quite familiar with the plight of many citizens who are addicted to drugs as well as with overloaded emergency rooms.

I have been in a number of them, and health care legislation was mentioned earlier by a colleague. As we discuss the impact of drug addicts and their needs in emergency rooms, we need to sort out those that have absolutely no emergency need but depend and descend upon emergency rooms because that is the only available source of health care, medical aid, that many citizens know.

One of our problems in California is the complete lack of an adequate, effective community-based mental health program. In 1969 when the liberals and the conservatives in the legislature banded together in the Short-Lanterman-Petris bill to save money and to make sure that Aunt Minnie wasn't incarcerated in a mental institution. They destroyed one of the best mental health programs in America and never funded the programs in California.

And so we need to not only deal with the supply end of the drug problem but to deal with the demand, whether it be through education or various types of health programs to end the addiction.

Mr. TOWNS. Thank you very much, Congressman Horn.

At this time, I would like to call our first witness, the Honorable Charles Rangel, the Dean of the New York delegation, that is "Dean" because of service, not in years of age.

He is a member of the powerful House Ways and Means Committee and the former chairman of the House Select Committee on Narcotics Abuse.

We are particularly pleased to have you appear before the subcommittee, Congressman Rangel. Recognizing your relationship in terms of your being in charge of the emergency room caucus, knowing how involved you have been in the subject down through the years, we would like to welcome you to the subcommittee; and you may proceed in any way you would like. Your entire testimony will be included in the record. If you want to summarize, feel free to do so.

Mr. RANGEL. Thank you, Mr. Chairman. And I do ask the consent of this committee to have my full statement in the record.

Mr. TOWNS. No objection, so moved.

STATEMENT OF HON. CHARLES B. RANGEL, A REPRESENTATIVE IN CONGRESS FROM THE STATE OF NEW YORK

Mr. RANGEL. Mr. Chairman, Mr. Schiff, my classmate, counsel, Mr. Mica. I hope New York City treated you and your family in a manner in which you are accustomed.

Mr. Horn.

This is a great honor for me to lead off the testimony on such a sensitive and important subject that you are taking up. I only hope that it gets the recognition and the publicity that it deserves. I have said that when one looks at the drug problem in the United

States of America, I cannot think of anything closer to a threat to our national security than drugs.

We normally go to our young people when it is time to defend the country and the things we believe in. The one thing that is being rejected more than ever are those who are dependent on alcohol and drugs. When we think about the largest problem that our Nation faces in terms of ever-increasing budget expenditures, it has to be our health problem; and drugs are hemorrhaging the cost that we pay there.

When you think about other costs that local and State governments have you see that we are spending $20 billion keeping young people in jail and another $20 billion for the jails that are coming online. And in our great city, Mr. Chairman, of New York, we pay $60,000 a year keeping someone in jail. National statistics show that 70 percent of them are going to return in 3 to 5 years.

So, it really doesn't make any difference which part of this problem we touch first. All of us working together have to come up with some kind of plan if we are going to have American youth to believe that, as our country recovers, at least somehow included in that great dream is improving the quality of life for themselves, their families and the communities.

When you take a look as to the impact of drug addiction on our emergency wards, it is absolutely unbelievable the nightmares that our doctors and nurses are going through.

When you see the relationship between drug addiction and kidney failure and the people that come in, even those that are on dialysis machines, drug addicts with a drug lifestyle disrupting not only the professional service that is given but also disrupting the services that are being rendered to people who don't have these alcohol and drug problems.

The most expensive health care that one can ever expect to pay is that care that is given in the hospitals. For every child that is born addicted to drugs, in New York City it costs $5,000 a day to treat that child. If the drug addict comes in and is diagnosed with tuberculosis, it is closer to $18,000 a day because of the new equipment that is necessary for hospitals to have to contain this new strand of tuberculosis in order that it does not contaminate a hospital.

Most of the hospitals in New York that have emergency rooms are affiliated with teaching hospitals. We have the best teaching hospitals in the world. Why? Because once you serve in our emergency room, there are no medical problems that you will not be able to resolve. So we have more than our share of doctors, even though, on a daily basis, they are really being burned out.

You have in my report the DAWN information which indicates an increase in the number of cases coming into emergency rooms that are drug related. Forget those figures. It is far more than ever is reported because doctors don't have the time to take urine specimen and check out whether or not the patient that arrives is on drugs or if the injury is drug related.

Is it drug related when we see the hundreds of cases pouring into our hospitals of gunshot wounds of dealers that are shooting each other out on the streets? Is it related when people come in with trauma, with heart trouble, with kidney failure, with strokes, all because they have misjudged the amount of drugs that the body could digest?

Home nurses and doctors have had to go through even the violence that is experienced with people who are completely out of control as they arrive in the emergency rooms.

I chair, as the chairman pointed out, the emergency room caucus. These doctors and nurses are not asking for more money. They feel it is a privilege to be able to serve in hospitals and in emergency rooms. But they say they just don't have enough people to give the quality of care that human beings deserve when they get into these rooms because of the length of hours that interns generally are required to spend but because of the number of cases that are pouring into these rooms because of the increase, in the inner cities especially, of drug use. It is not getting any better, Mr. Chairman.

We have no foreign policy at all as relates to where 98 percent of the drugs are being grown, that is the cocaine out of Peru. We don't even have an assistant Secretary of State confirmed for this area. Just yesterday the Senate took up the question of confirming the drug czar, but you haven't heard from any Secretary of Health—including the one we have now—ever speak about really what is hemorrhaging our health delivery system. The most expensive part of it is hospitals. The most expensive part of hospital care is in the emergency room.

When last has anyone on this panel ever heard a Secretary of Education include in his portfolio the fact that we are going to have to educate our children that their lives are worth more drug free than they are on the streets of our inner cities? They just don't talk about it.

When last has anyone on this panel ever heard any Secretary of State think it was important enough to mention the countries that we do business with that really allow drugs to pour across their borders into the international community and yet we don't upon even offend anybody by raising it?

And what are the big issues we have now? It is the North American Free Trade Agreement. Do you know that Ambassador Carla Hills said it would be offensive to talk about drugs with our friends in Mexico. Of the drugs, no matter where they come from, 70 percent cross the Mexican border. Isn't it logical to believe that if we are going to have more trade with Mexico that there would be the opportunity of more drugs to come into the United States?

What I was asking of Chairman Rostenkowski and our committee was that we be more vigilant in terms of drugs coming into the United States, to have more border patrols and more customs officers.

I am saying that you really may have a tiger by the tail, because as the Nation starts talking about more coverage and more expenses, you guys have really found out where the most per capita expenses as it relates to health treatment really is; our Nations hospitals and our Nation's emergency rooms.

The select committee, as you know, has formed a congressional caucus to deal with this problem. The chairman certainly sits on that caucus. We have a lot of the information already researched that we are prepared to turn over to this committee in support of the fine work that you are getting involved in.

I say, how could you possibly talk about comprehensive health insurance for the Nation without stepping aside, looking back, and seeing what drugs and alcohol are really costing us?

So I am excited about where this committee is going to take this subject matter. I stand ready with so many Members of Congress to support you in this work.

Thank you so much for the opportunity to give my views, and I will be glad to answer any questions if you have some.

[The prepared statement of Mr. Rangel follows:]

85-837 O - 95 - 2

INCREASED DRUG ABUSE AND THE
IMPACT ON THE NATION'S EMERGENCY
ROOMS

CONGRESSMAN CHARLES B.RANGEL

TESTIMONY BEFORE THE SUBCOMMITTEE
ON HUMAN RESOURCES
AND
INTERGOVERNMENTAL RELATIONS

MAY 26,1993

GOOD MORNING CHAIRMAN TOWNS AND MEMBERS OF THE SUBCOMMITTEE ON HUMAN RESOURCES AND INTERGOVERNMENTAL RELATIONS. IT IS A PLEASURE TO APPEAR BEFORE YOU TODAY TO ADDRESS THE VERY IMPORTANT TOPIC OF ASSESSING INCREASED DRUG ABUSE AND THE IMPACT ON THE NATION'S EMERGENCY ROOMS. YOU WILL ALSO HEAR FROM OTHER MEDICAL AND LAW ENFORCEMENT EXPERTS TODAY ON THIS TOPIC AND I COMMEND YOU FOR FOCUSING THE RESOURCES OF YOUR SUBCOMMITTEE ON THIS ISSUE.

AS YOU KNOW, UNTIL RECENTLY I CHAIRED THE CONGRESSIONAL SELECT COMMITTEE ON NARCOTICS ABUSE AND CONTROL WHICH THROUGH VARIOUS HEARINGS AND INVESTIGATIVE WORK GATHERED INFORMATION ON MANY ISSUES INCLUDING THE INCREASE OF DRUG ABUSE. MUCH OF THAT INFORMATION IS STILL TIMELY TODAY EVEN THOUGH THE ACTUAL WORK WAS CARRIED OUT OVER THE PAST FEW YEARS. MUCH OF THIS INFORMATION WILL BE FURTHER DOCUMENTED BY UPDATED INFORMATION THAT I INTEND TO GATHER IN THE FUTURE THROUGH OUR NEWLY CREATED CONGRESSIONAL NARCOTICS ABUSE AND CONTROL CAUCUS WHICH WAS RECENTLY AUTHORIZED AS AN LSO BY HOUSE ADMINISTRATION.

FROM BACKGROUND INFORMATION ALREADY AVAILABLE FROM OUR PAST WORK WE HAVE SEEN A CLEAR PICTURE EMERGE ABOUT THE SERIOUS IMPACT INCREASED DRUG USAGE IS HAVING ON HOSPITAL EMERGENCY ROOMS AND THE QUALITY OF CARE IN OUR NATION'S PUBLIC HOSPITALS. ALTHOUGH SOME SURVEYS INDICATE THAT CASUAL DRUG USE HAS DECLINED, FREQUENT AND HARDCORE USE OF HEROIN, AND COCAINE REMAIN HIGH AND APPEAR TO BE INCREASING. THE CONTINUING DRUG CRISIS IS OVERBURDENING THE NATION'S EMERGENCY MEDICAL SERVICES. DRUG OVERDOSES AND PHYSICAL INJURIES RESULTING FROM DRUG-RELATED VIOLENCE ARE CONTRIBUTING SUBSTANTIALLY TO THE REDUCED QUALITY OF CARE PROVIDED BY MANY EMERGENCY ROOMS. THE DRUG CRISIS IS STRAINING A SYSTEM ALREADY DETERIORATING IN THE FACE OF THE AIDS EPIDEMIC AND THE MEDICAL DEMANDS OF 37 MILLION UNINSURED AMERICANS AND ANOTHER 100 MILLION UNDERINSURED PEOPLE WHO OFTEN HAVE NO CHOICE BUT TO RELY ON THE NATION'S EMERGENCY MEDICAL SYSTEM FOR THEIR PRIMARY HEALTH CARE NEEDS.

THE IMPACT OF INCREASED HARDCORE DRUG USE ON HOSPITAL EMERGENCY ROOMS IS CLEARLY EVIDENT IN THE RISING LEVELS OF DRUG OVERDOSE CASES. WITH THE ADVENT OF THE CRACK COCAINE EPIDEMIC IN THE MID 1980'S, COCAINE-RELATED HOSPITAL EMERGENCY ROOM EPISODES SKYROCKETED. HEROIN-RELATED EPISODES ALSO INCREASED SIGNIFICANTLY. AFTER DECLINING FOR

A BRIEF PERIOD IN 1989 AND 1990, COCAINE AND HEROIN HOSPITAL EMERGENCY ROOM EPISODES RETURNED TO THEIR EARLIER RECORD LEVELS IN 1992.

WE RECENTLY HAD THIS ISSUE PUT SQUARELY IN FRONT OF US AGAIN IN THE APRIL 1993 RELEASE BY THE DEPARTMENT OF HEALTH AND HUMAN SERVICES OF THE STATISTICAL INFORMATION THEY GATHERED THROUGH D.A.W.N.,THE DRUG ABUSE WARNING NETWORK. D.A.W.N. COLLECTS DATA ON THE CONSEQUENCES OF DRUG ABUSE BY MEASURING DRUG RELATED EPISODES AND MENTIONS IN A NATIONALLY REPRESENTATIVE SAMPLE OF HOSPITAL EMERGENCY ROOMS IN THE UNITED STATES. I SHARED THIS INFORMATION WITH OTHER MEMBERS THROUGH MY APRIL 27,1993 DEAR COLLEAGUE LETTER AND WILL ALSO SUBMIT IT FOR THE RECORD AT THIS HEARING. IN MY LETTER I POINTED OUT THAT DESPITE IMPROVEMENTS IN CASUAL DRUG USE, THE LATEST GOVERNMENT STATISTICS IN EMERGENCY ROOM VISITS SHOW SHARP INCREASES AMONG THE HEAVIEST USERS. THE NUMBER OF COCAINE USERS SEEKING EMERGENCY ROOM HELP INCREASED TO NEARLY 31,000 IN 1992, 8.2% OVER THE SAME PERIOD IN 1991. HEROIN RELATED PROBLEMS SHOWED A DRAMATIC INCREASE OF NEARLY 30%,UP TO MORE THAN 13,000 VISITS LAST SUMMER FROM 10,000 THE PREVIOUS YEAR.

NOT ONLY DO THESE NUMBERS SHOW THE INCREASE IN DRUG USAGE BUT THEY WERE DEVELOPED FROM THE VERY HOSPITAL EMERGENCY ROOMS THAT ARE A FOCUS OF THIS HEARING. INCREASED DRUG TRAFFIC IN OUR NATION'S URBAN AREAS AND THE COMPETITION FOR LUCRATIVE DRUG MARKETS HAS SPAWNED AN UPWARD SPIRAL OF DRUG-RELATED VIOLENCE THAT IS WREAKING HAVOC ON MANY INNER CITY TRAUMA CENTERS.

•IN ONE OAKLAND, CALIFORNIA, HOSPITAL, THE NUMBER OF CASES INVOLVING GUNSHOT AND STAB WOUNDS INCREASED 33 PERCENT FROM 1987 TO 1989.

•THE USE OF AUTOMATIC WEAPONS, A TRADEMARK OF VIOLENT DRUG GANGS AND DEALERS, IS COMPOUNDING THE NUMBER AND SEVERITY OF INJURIES SEEN IN EMERGENCY ROOMS AND TRAUMA CENTERS. IN THE COOK COUNTY HOSPITAL, FOR EXAMPLE, GUNSHOT VICTIMS WITH MORE THAN ONE WOUND INCREASED FROM 5% IN 1984 TO 20% IN 1988.

•ACCORDING TO ONE ESTIMATE BY A FORMER ADVISER TO PRESIDENT BUSH, THE UNITED STATES SPENT $4.4 BILLION TO TREAT GUNSHOT WOUND VICTIMS IN 1990.

DRUG-RELATED OVERDOSES REPORTED THROUGH D.A.W.N. AND TRAUMA CASES RESULTING FROM DRUG VIOLENCE ARE ONLY THE TIP OF THE ICEBERG IN TERMS OF THE IMPACT OF DRUGS ON THE NATION'S HOSPITAL EMERGENCY ROOMS. TESTIMONY BEFORE THE SELECT COMMITTEE ON NARCOTICS BY EMERGENCY ROOM PHYSICIANS WAS UNEQUIVOCAL THAT MANY PATIENTS WHO COME TO EMERGENCY ROOMS FOR PROBLEMS THAT ARE CAUSALLY RELATED TO DRUGS ARE OVERLOOKED BY CURRENT DATA SYSTEMS, SUCH AS D.A.W.N. THAT ONLY COUNT THE MOST OVERT CASE OF DRUG-RELATED INJURY OR ILLNESS. FOR EXAMPLE, EMERGENCY ROOM VISITS BY IV DRUG USERS WHO NEED TREATMENT FOR KIDNEY, LUNG AND HEART AILMENTS OR AIDS COMPLICATIONS RELATED TO THEIR DRUG USE ARE NOT COUNTED AS DRUG-RELATED VISITS. ALSO, GIVEN THE TIME CONSTRAINTS AND PRESSURES OF MANY LARGE URBAN HOSPITAL EMERGENCY ROOMS, DOCTORS TESTIFIED THAT THEY ONLY DEAL WITH AND DOCUMENT THE MOST EVIDENT PROBLEM. THEY DON'T HAVE THE TIME TO NOTE ON THE CHART THAT DRUGS WERE A FACTOR. AS A RESULT, THE DOCTORS SAID, MANY DRUG-RELATED EMERGENCY CASES THAT INVOLVE OBSTETRICS, TRAUMA OR OTHER MEDICAL PROBLEMS ARE OFTEN OVERLOOKED BY EXISTING SURVEILLANCE SYSTEMS.

IN MY VIEW THIS DATA IS DISTURBING NEWS NOT ONLY FOR THE POOR INNER CITY COMMUNITIES BUT ALSO FOR THE MIDDLE INCOME FAMILIES WHO RELY ON INCREASINGLY BURDENED HOSPITAL

EMERGENCY ROOM SERVICES. THE RISE IN FREQUENCY OF DRUG-RELATED EMERGENCY ROOM VISITS ALSO REPRESENTS THE CONTINUATION OF A TREND WHICH BEGAN IN 1991 AFTER A BRIEF PERIOD OF DECLINE. IT IS CLEAR THAT NOT ONLY IS THERE AN INCREASE IN DRUG USAGE BUT THE INSTANT TREATMENT IS BEING PROVIDED BY HOSPITAL EMERGENCY ROOMS ALREADY OVERBURDENED IN THEIR EFFORTS TO EFFECTIVELY HANDLE THE HOMICIDES,ASSAULTS AND OTHER VIOLENT CASES COMING THROUGH THEIR DOORS.

BECAUSE OF THE INCREASED IMPACT OF DRUG-RELATED CASES ON URBAN HOSPITAL EMERGENCY ROOMS, I JOINED WITH REP. HENRY WAXMAN SEVERAL YEARS AGO TO SPONSOR LEGISLATION TO ALLEVIATE THIS PROBLEM. OUR BILL AUTHORIZED GRANTS TO HOSPITAL TRAUMA CENTERS THAT HAVE INCURRED SUBSTANTIAL UNCOMPENSATED COSTS IN PROVIDING EMERGENCY ROOM CARE TO VICTIMS OF DRUG-RELATED VIOLENCE. IN 1988, U.S. HOSPITALS LOST AN ESTIMATED $1 BILLION PROVIDING TRAUMA CARE TO THOSE WITHOUT THE MEANS TO PAY. MOST HOSPITALS REPORT ANNUAL LOSES OF $1 MILLION TO $6 MILLION IN THEIR TRAUMA CENTER OPERATIONS. LAST YEAR, A VERSION OF OUR LEGISLATION AUTHORIZING $100 MILLION ANNUALLY FOR GRANTS TO TRAUMA CENTERS IMPACTED BY DRUG-RELATED VIOLENCE WAS ENACTED AS PART OF S. 1306, THE ADAMHA REORGANIZATION ACT (P. L. 102-321). UNFORTUNATELY, HOWEVER, CURRENT BUDGET CONSTRAINTS HAVE MADE IT IMPOSSIBLE TO APPROPRIATE FUNDS FOR THE

RELIEF SO URGENTLY NEEDED BY MANY OF OUR NATION'S HARD-PRESSED EMERGENCY ROOMS.

MANY OF THE ISSUES RELATED TO EMERGENCY ROOM SERVICES AND DRUG ABUSE MUST BE ADDRESSED THROUGH THE RECOMMENDATIONS THAT WILL BE COMING FROM PRESIDENT CLINTON'S HEALTH REFORM PACKAGE. I SHOULD ALSO POINT OUT THAT IN LINE WITH THIS ISSUE I WILL,ALONG WITH COLUMBIA UNIVERSITY PRESIDENT MICHAEL I. SOVERN,BE SPONSORING AT HARLEM HOSPITAL CENTER ON JUNE 7th AND 8th,A CONFERENCE ON "HEALTH CARE IN UNDERSERVED URBAN AMERICA:IMPLICATIONS FOR NATIONAL HEALTH REFORM"WHICH WILL TAKE INTO ACCOUNT EMERGENCY ROOM AND OTHER URBAN HEALTH CARE ISSUES.

IN MY ESTIMATION WE HAVE CLEAR EVIDENCE THAT DRUG ABUSE CONTINUES IN OUR COUNTRY AND WE MUST BE VIGILANT IN ADDRESSING OUR PREVENTION,LAW ENFORCEMENT AND TREATMENT NEED.BUT WE MUST ALSO BE AWARE THAT HOW WE HANDLE OUR FOREIGN POLICY CAN RESULT IN THE INCREASE OF DRUGS COMING INTO OUR COMMUNITIES AND EVENTUALLY SENDING CLIENTS TO OUR EMERGENCY ROOMS. ONE CLEAR EXAMPLE OF OUR NEED FOR VIGILANCE WAS AGAIN A FRONT PAGE STORY IN THE MONDAY MAY 24,1993 EDITION OF THE NEW YORK TIMES WHICH DISCUSSED AN ISSUE THAT I ATTEMPTED ON NUMEROUS OCCASIONS TO BRING TO THE ATTENTION OF THE CONGRESS AS WELL AS FORMER U.S. TRADE

REPRESENTATIVE CARLA HILL. THIS IS MY CONCERN ABOUT THE NAFTA TREATY WHICH,IN MY VIEW,IS AN OPEN INVITATION TO FURTHER TRAFFICKING OF DRUGS INTO OUR COUNTRY. AS COVERED IN THIS ARTICLE,WHICH I WILL SUBMIT FOR THE RECORD,ACCORDING TO AN INTELLIGENCE REPORT TO THE STATE DEPARTMENT,"UNITED STATES INTELLIGENCE AND LAW ENFORCEMENT OFFICIALS, WARN THAT COCAINE SMUGGLERS WORKING WITH COLOMBIAN DRUG CARTELS ARE STARTING TO SET UP FACTORIES,WAREHOUSES AND TRUCKING COMPANIES IN MEXICO TO EXPLOIT THE FLOOD OF CROSS-BORDER COMMERCE EXPECTED UNDER THE NORTH AMERICAN FREE TRADE AGREEMENT."

WHILE TO SOME THE DRUG FIELDS OF MEXICO MIGHT SEEM TO BE A LONG WAY FROM THE HOSPITAL EMERGENCY ROOMS IN OUR URBAN AND RURAL COMMUNITIES BELIEVE THERE IS A REAL CONNECTION.WE NEED TO BE AWARE OF THIS TIMELY WARNING AS WE CONTINUE OUR DISCUSSIONS ABOUT NAFTA AND INSURE THAT DURING THESE DISCUSSIONS THAT THE DRUG ABUSE CONCERN IS PART OF THE DIALOGUE.

MR. CHAIRMAN THANK YOU FOR ALLOWING ME TIME THIS MORNING TO SHARE MY VIEWS WITH YOU AND THE SUBCOMMITTEE NOT ONLY ON THE TOPIC OF DRUG INCREASE AND EMERGENCY ROOM IMPACT BUT ALSO LISTENING TO MY GENERAL CONCERN ABOUT THE NEED TO BE EVER VIGILANT IN OUR DEVELOPMENT OF NATIONAL

DRUG POLICY. I'M HAPPY TO REPORT THAT YESTERDAY I HAD THE OPPORTUNITY TO INTRODUCE MR. LEE P. BROWN TO THE SENATE JUDICIARY COMMITTEE AS PRESIDENT CLINTON'S NOMINEE TO BE THE DRUG CZAR. I FEEL CONFIDENT THAT MR. BROWN WILL BE AN ASSET TO THE PRESIDENT'S TEAM AND WILL FOCUS ON OVERALL DRUG ABUSE AND HEALTH ISSUES INCLUDING THE IMPACT OF DRUG USE INCREASES ON EMERGENCY ROOM SERVICES.

I WILL RESPOND TO ANY QUESTIONS FROM YOU OR OTHER SUBCOMMITTEE MEMBERS.

Mr. TOWNS. Thank you very much Congressman Rangel for your outstanding testimony. It was very informative.

One of the problems that we hear from time to time is what is happening in some of our major cities. For instance, the drug problem that we now see in New York, in reference to the use of heroin, it will be 10 maybe 12 years before it reaches out to some of the other areas. Therefore, being that it is in New York, there is no need for them to get involved.

What can we do to sort of build allies and let people know that the problems in New York or the problems in Miami or the problems in many of our major cities around the Nation, will be in their areas as well.

What can we do to build support?

Mr. RANGEL. That is a hard job Mr. Chairman. I was prosecuting in the Federal courts drug traffickers when we had really organized crime syndicates.

I was saying in the 1960's that the heroin that was being poured into my Harlem district and happening in the black and poor communities throughout the country, that soon it would jump over the walls of the ghetto and go into other communities; and that did happen, as it did with cocaine.

But you know, our major problem today is not just the cocaine but the crack cocaine. The reason you find the explosion in the heroin that is being consumed is because drug addicts now find that the euphoria that you get from the crack is a fast high but it doesn't last that long.

On the other hand, the heroin is longer lasting. So they are smoking it instead of injecting it.

You will find that we are not increasing the number of heroin users that inject, but there is a sharp increase in the number of heroin users that smoke.

But why we cannot get the attention we deserve is because if you look at the evening news, one would think that the drug consumers in America were young black and Hispanic youth? The reason you get that perception is that these kids, uneducated, nothing to lose, are in the streets and really exposing themselves to being arrested and going to jail is no big deal to them.

They get free medical care, free meals, adult supervision, climate control, recreation, color TV, and self-esteem in dealing with their peers.

The truth of the matter is that 80 percent of the drugs that are consumed in America are by nonminority, affluent people. They know how to use drugs in a way that do not expose them to the dangers of arrest, you don't find America concerned about them. We don't even know the damage that is being done in our board rooms and our classrooms, on our transportation systems, in our air traffic controllers.

And, yet, minorities are not consuming 80 percent of the drugs that come into the United States.

Now, true, one of the things that we can do is say that if you ignore what is happening in the inner cities, if you ignore the high health rates, if you ignore the high crime rates, if you ignore the high costs of incarceration, ultimately, you are really—America is really losing.

Dick Darmen was able to prepare papers for our committee to show the result of the high cost of health care, crime, incarceration, loss of productivity, and loss of revenue that the drug problem costs $300 billion a year.

How in the heck are we going to be competitive if we go and say that we have over a million people locked up? They should be locked up in school. They should be locked up in work forces. They should be locked up learning how to do something to be productive. Their minds should be opened up to an alternative instead of a life of drugs, crime, and jail.

And so it would seem to me, Mr. Chairman, at least the approach that I have taken, we can't do it for humane reasons. Right now, we have to be concerned about capping entitlements. We cannot spend too much money on the aged and on the poor. But if we are so concerned about budget restrictions, reducing the deficit, why in God's name don't we talk about the emergency room costs that addicts are causing? The cost of keeping an addict in prison? The fact that if we are going to be productive and competitive, how do we tell the world that we have a million people locked up in jail and we have to compete with Japan and the European Common market.

Mr. Chairman, all of us have to try to get our message across in different ways. But being on the Ways and Means Committee, knowing that the Nation is concerned about excessive spending and heavy taxation, I have chosen to do what you are starting this hearing for, to say, how much is it costing you to do nothing about this serious problem?

Mr. TOWNS. Thank you very much, Mr. Rangel.

At this time I would yield to the ranking member, Congressman Schiff.

Mr. RANGEL. Buenos dias.

Mr. SCHIFF. I have the feeling whoever may be watching through the TV will laugh at my Spanish, but I will say buenos dias, because we are classmates in Spanish class.

Chairman Rangel, it is always a pleasure to listen to you and to hear your views from the body of experience that you bring with you, as you share your views with us as your colleagues.

I would like to ask about one particular issue and that is the issue of incarceration as it forms a part of our total approach. Even though I am a former prosecutor, I am also a former defense attorney. I have never believed that jails and prisons are the only solution to the problem.

Nevertheless, you made a statement I would like to pursue with you about our incarcerating people for being addicts. And it is simply my experience, in quite a number of years practicing in criminal justice, that I am just not aware that there are that many people in custody for simply being addicts. And when I use the word "simply," that is in the criminal law context, not demeaning the importance of the situation of someone being an addict.

But my experience with the system is that people who by and large are in custody for mere possession, again using this as a legal term, are normally given the opportunity for some kind of rehabilitation. And the people who are in custody either failed in that opportunity and did it again and again and again or more likely were traffickers.

It is my understanding that most of the people in custody relating to narcotics are there for trafficking in narcotics, not using narcotics.

Mr. RANGEL. I agree with you. Either I misspoke or I was misunderstood. Of the people in urban jails 80 percent are there for drug-related crimes. It is certainly not just walking around with drugs in their pocket.

But let's think about it, Mr. Former prosecutor——

Mr. SCHIFF. And former defense attorney. I will take both titles.

Mr. RANGEL [continuing]. Isn't it true that most of these addicts are not only unemployed but unemployable?

Mr. SCHIFF. Are you asking for my view of the situation? I will be glad to share it with you.

Mr. RANGEL. That was rhetorical because I assume that your reply would be yes.

So if you are buying drugs on the streets, and this is the difference between—and I don't want to say that it is a stark racial thing but a stark economic thing. Those that are working and can pay for their drugs are not in jail. Those who are not working, who are addicts, commit crimes in order to get the money, what is their crime? You say dealing in drugs. Give me a break.

These illiterates, addicts, sell these drugs to support their habit. Are they breaking the law? Yes. Should they be arrested? Yes. Should they go to jail? Yes. I am for swift law enforcement.

I am saying that under the mandatory penalties, a kid that sells drugs twice faces a mandatory 10 years, next time 30 years. What are we proving by putting a kid in jail that long?

I am saying that we should review the sentencing law; and if it is a first offender, put him in a work camp; teach him how to paint, how to be an electrician, be a carpenter, so at least when he gets out he has an alternative to going back to drugs.

The experience that I have when a guy is arrested for drugs, he has lost his job, his friends; he is unemployable; he goes back on the block and the only people that talk to him are the peers; the graduates of the jail system. He goes back to drugs.

Mr. SCHIFF. Let me separate that out. With respect to the first time, nonviolent offender—what about the individual who is doing it for a fast buck? The individual—and I run into this a great number of times in the nonminority community especially. It is presented almost like this is an alternative that the administration should consider to financing college education. Young individuals get offered money to deliver drugs to one point or another. They are not addicts.

They simply made the decision that this was easier money and faster money than getting it through a law-abiding manner of attaining funds. It has nothing to do with their being addicts because they are not addicts.

Do you consider those people also in the group of individuals whom we should otherwise treat as simple nonviolent offenders?

Mr. RANGEL. I certainly do. There is no equal justice under the law. I prosecuted, and I know I have never prosecuted a money launderer or a banker. I never prosecuted the people who sell these kids the foreign cars. All of them are violating the law.

You don't read in the papers about how the affluent people who are really the financiers of the enormous international drug trafficking, they are never arrested. They are never brought into court, and they are never given sentences.

Now, if you really think that you should not take another view of these nonaddict traffickers, I would say you ought to put them in categories.

If a guy is a big-time trafficker and he is making tens and thousands of dollars, put him in jail, throw away the key, and forget about him because we have to really not only punish him but we need something to serve as a deterrent.

But if you agree with me that over 90 percent of the kids that are out there selling are illiterate, dropouts unemployable, and they are willing to get on the street to risk their lives because they do, you know that, to make $1,000 a day or more and they are so stupid really that in New York City—and in many of your urban communities—when they get arrested, they have suitcases full of money. Why? They don't know how to launder it. They don't know how to go to fancy restaurants and order things. They don't know how to go to a tailor. They don't know how to go to a travel agent and have a trip. They don't know many of the alternatives in our community, having left school and not having job opportunities.

In these committees you will find that the unemployment rate for teenagers are 2, 3, 4 times the national average.

The real answer, Mr. Schiff, has to be: Did the kid really have an opportunity and have reason to believe that they could make it in a noncriminal way? Or is society kind of willing to spend $60,000 to keep him in jail, but less than $6,000 a year to keep him in school.

I am saying this—and let me conclude because I am talking too long—I am working with Mr. Payne very closely with the Haitian Government and President Aristide to get him back into Haiti and the chairman. One of the things that we have to do is negotiate how much money the international community is going to put up and also the conditions in which he is to return.

One of the key points was the issue of amnesty. Normally, everyone knows what amnesty means; but when diplomats talk about it, it means 15, 10, 20 different things. How dare you offer me amnesty, I didn't do anything. But the question of amnesty for the bums in the army for the people that are repressing the people never came up. Why? Because the President decided that these people never really had a choice. They were poor, hungry, illiterate. He wants them to give up the guns, get an education, and rebuild Haiti. I am listening to him, and I am saying if it is good enough for the Haitian soldiers who have committed crimes against their people, then it should be good enough for the million people or close to that in terms of isolating the violent criminals, to give our young people a chance to be educated and to give them an opportunity.

If we drop the ball on that, Mr. Schiff, if after we have taught them a trade, given them an opportunity for public service and still they go to have a life of crime, I think we should be very severe with them.

Mr. SCHIFF. Thank you Mr. Rangel.

I yield back, Mr. Chairman.

Mr. TOWNS. Let me note that we have been joined by Congressman Payne from Newark, NJ.

And I would pass over him at this time, and I call on Congressman Mica.

Mr. MICA. Thank you, Mr. Chairman.

Mr. Rangel, there is probably no one who is better identified with a continuous, nonstop effort to deal with the problem of drug abuse in the Congress than you. I commend you on your many years of work.

We had a meeting not too long ago with all the different folks from the enforcement side, a dinner meeting. And, unfortunately, I think there were only four Members of Congress that came to that meeting. And I was really saddened to see that. I am saddened to see that you are still the sort of lone stranger leading this force when you point out very well that this is the biggest social problem facing the country.

And for African Americans or black Americans, you have a Bosnia practically every weekend in some of the cities here. I don't return here one weekend without reading the Washington Post and seeing the genocide of black males from 15 to 40.

And you point out the social inequities. The question is, what do we do about it? As I said before, when I worked on the Senate side, we worked on the enforcement side. And it is true that you have to keep the pressure on these producing countries and trafficking countries. But I am wondering now if we really don't need to do more in education and prevention.

And I know we have limited resources and that is one reason why I discussed briefly before you got here the impact of narcotics in our society. The home, the school, and the church or synagogue don't have the impact that they used to have on young people.

And I have identified one of the great resources of the Federal Government is the airwaves, with television. It impacts people in what they buy, whether it is soap powder or the kind of clothes they wear or how they dance or whatever. And we have been looking at this draft legislation that deals with requiring as part of the public service requirement for a television stations, that they devote at least 5 percent of their commercial time to drug education and prevention.

My question is: Do you think that this is a viable alternative? You see the changes we have made just in the past 12 or 15 years say on smoking. The back of this room would probably have been filled with smokers, 12 or 15 years ago, and people are not smoking—it is still a health problem. But we have educated people a bit.

So I am wondering if we can't use an inexpensive medium, which is free—there is a public requirement for television stations to broadcast—to help educate folks. Just soliciting your opinion?

Mr. RANGEL. Well, there are varied opinions, and I always think everything that you can do helps. I am a little outraged when I hear people in the Clinton administration saying that they are going to give more emphasis to one area of the budget than the other, when really you never had a program to determine what the budget should be.

So to take the other President's budget and say that you are going to reorganize; and not knowing what worked and what didn't work, I really think it is premature.

When it comes to television, sure, it has an overwhelming impression on people's habits. I think, to a large extent, it is responsible for the reduction in drug consumption among the affluent Americans. The problem that you have, as I see it, is that even when it comes to smoking, the people who have stopped smoking or won't smoke are people who are concerned about their bodies and their lives. I would bet that they are the most educated people in the America and recognized that smoking is bad for them, and it is not even worth the little enjoyment they get out of it.

In addition to that, they would be people that really got something to look forward to in life, and they want to live because they know that life for them should be getting better, seeing their kids grow up and go to college and to become grandparents.

It is enough for people to say, hey, it is not worth it. I really think that we are going to have to go beyond the television and to make certain that our young people have an alternative to a life of drugs. Sometimes I walk down the streets of Lenox Avenue and addicts are lying in front of clinics for methadone congratulating me for the job that I am doing in the fight on drugs. I say, you are putting me on? Why are you congratulating me? They say, hey it is all over for me. I have pain, and I need drugs, and it is all over anyway.

But whatever you can do to prevent the young people from doing it, I would support. While I support anything that you can do to get the television industry to be more responsive—and they have made a real tremendous contribution already—it is good.

But if you can do it in that classroom, if you can have a kid believe that doing drugs may disrupt their ability to be employable, to make a contribution, to get a paycheck, that the family may reject them, that the church and community may reject them for doing drugs, to me, that is why it is important.

The fact is, Mr. Mica, we haven't done anything there. We have—no Secretary of Education has gone beyond some coloring book in saying that we are mandating. If you mandate saying the pledge of allegiance to the flag, if you mandate the singing of the Star Spangled Banner, then we should mandate that you have an opportunity to be a productive citizen and serve your country.

Mr. TOWNS. Thank you.

Congressman Horn—I'm sorry. It is Congressman Payne.

Mr. PAYNE. Thank you very much, Mr. Chairman.

Let me congratulate you and commend you for your leadership on having this very important hearing today. And also let me commend you for last week when you had Mayor Dinkens, an outstanding person from the community in elected positions from around the country to come before your committee to talk about the problems of urban America and the problems that confront us and the problems that we need to resolve for us to put America back on track and move toward a society that has freedom and justice for all.

Let me also commend Mr. Rangel, the most nationally renowned expert on the question of substance abuse, who has done such a

85-837 O - 95 - 3

yeoman's job leading the fight. And long before I came to Congress, I knew about Mr. Rangel and the work that he did in this arena.

I won't ask any questions at this time, but would like to commend both you and him for this hearing. And I would reserve the opportunity to make a statement following Mr. Rangel's completed testimony and simply before the next witness, if you will permit it.

Mr. TOWNS. With no objection, so moved.

Let me thank the gentleman for his kind words.

Congressman Horn.

Mr. HORN. Thank you, Mr. Chairman. The gentleman from New York's eloquence is well known and your knowledge in particular. I have admired, as I told you privately the other day, what you have done over the years.

Let me ask you about the related areas that seem to be changing, and I would like your perspective on it.

In California, we obviously have very serious drug problems just as any urban area in the city of Los Angeles and every city in the State what has changed in 20 years, not only what you mentioned on the crack situation, and we have approximately 80,000 crack babies a year born in California. And you can imagine what the schools will be like in 3, 4, 5 years.

But what has changed is where individuals used to come over our borders, either the Canadian border to Detroit or the Mexican border to the southwest and looking for job opportunities, but now they seem to be coming over more and more with drugs.

Is that your perception? You are an exhibit in this area. The data seems to be changing in that regard.

Mr. RANGEL. Yes. Really not as drug dealers. Just enough to think that they could sell it, and that was to get started in society.

It is unfortunately true that a lot of—they call them mules—Mexicans cross the border. People tell them, take this; here is $25; when you get there, somebody will greet you. If they get arrested and go to jail, it is no great loss. They have hundreds of mules.

It is true that poor folks and those seeking a better way of life, they don't realize sometimes the dangerous job that they are doing.

Mr. HORN. In essence, they might as well be smuggling atomic bombs in in terms of the damage they are doing. But for some reason, we can't seem to control our borders and face up to the problem. That is one way to get at the supply.

Mr. RANGEL. Mr. Horn, I have stayed in hot water with our trade negotiators with Mexico and it is not as though I am against free trade. I truly believe if America is going to be competitive, that we have to consolidate our resources in this hemisphere if we are going to compete with Europe and Asia.

But the major problem we have, Mr. Horn, is in the State Department. It is this uncanny belief that you can't offend foreigners; you cannot talk with them in a way about what they are doing to you. Each time you approach the situation, somebody in the State Department is going to talk about how sensitive they are. I don't understand it because, as you say, they are bringing bombs across our borders; and we should at least be able to say, listen, we want to do trade with you, and we are going to put up people on our side in order to make certain that we have some protection. What are you going to do on your side of the border to make certain that your people are screened before they come across?

But again if Carla Hills told me once, she told me a million times, "Mr. Rangel, that is apples and oranges; you are talking about illicit trade. We are talking about legal trade. And we cannot do this to the Mexicans because if we did, we will single them out; and we are not doing it to any other country." I said, "Why don't we do it to the other countries? Why don't we do it to Canada and tell everybody that we are frightened to death that this is eating away at the very heart of our country?"

I tell you one thing, the breath of fresh air is that Lee Brown truly believes that he has an agreement with this Secretary of State to be tough on these countries, cooperatives with these countries, and to come up with some plans. Lucky for us, Lee Brown is the only candidate for this type of work with the Federal Government that I know that has no political ambitions. He was begged to take the job. He brings his own credibility, and he really believes he can make a contribution.

I am excited about the opportunity, even though he starts off late, that, as a Cabinet official with the full support of the President of the United States, he can tell the President, "I am trying to do the best I can with Peru, but the Secretary says I can't talk about it." He points out where we are not really getting the cooperation that we deserve. I could go on and on.

But the last thing is that we have these Dominicans who have the best connection in the world with the Colombians. Now, they come to the Dominican Republic. They create the drug traffickers. They have communities in the Dominican Republic where the youngsters are trained just to come to the United States to sell drugs. They have some magic number in pesos that if they get a quarter of a million dollars, they quit and retire and go back home.

But they don't mind risking their lives because there are about 400 bodies a year that leave my district.

Mr. WASHINGTON. Heights community that are shipped back to one or two towns in the Dominican Republic. How do they get into my district so easily? They go to Puerto Rico. I am not saying that all Latinos look alike, but the language and everything else, once they get to Puerto Rico, they come into the United States. Are you an American citizen? And they say, si. Si; and they come into the United States.

It is wrong not to put the resources in Puerto Rico to stop it. And it is wrong that they are coming into Kennedy Airport with drugs, and we don't say that this is hemorrhaging our criminal justice system as well as our quality of life.

Mr. HORN. Do you think we need more border patrol? Is there a role for the American military to, at least, maybe without guns or whatever, be maneuvering on our borders or what?

Mr. RANGEL. We have to do all of those things. We have to hit our schools and make certain there is treatment and take another look at what we are doing with those in jails.

We have to let those countries that are doing business with us know that there is a narcotics problem.

We don't have any more communists to shoot down. Where is all this technology. If we can detect flying objects in the air, why can't we detect what is crossing our borders? Why is it that with all the military that we have, that we can't assign them—I mean, when I was on maneuvers in the Army, they had me in some mountain area looking for duds because it was used for artillery. It was not a very pleasant job. I think it would be far more pleasant to have the maneuvers on our borders to act like we are being invaded and check those people that are not coming into our country at checkpoints. They are there.

There is no great communist threat. I don't think we are going to Bosnia, so there is something for them to do.

Mr. HORN. I would be glad to join you in a bipartisan letter to that effect to the President and the Secretary of State and the Secretary of Defense.

Mr. RANGEL. Terrific. I knew if I came here, I would pick up something.

Mr. TOWNS. At this time, I yield to the gentleman from New Jersey.

Mr. PAYNE. Thank you.

I wouldn't want to detain the witness any longer, and I could give my statement after he leaves.

Mr. TOWNS. Let me thank the witness. I think you are so right. We need a comprehensive approach to the problem. And I would like to thank you for all the years and time that you put into it.

As I listened to you with all the problems that we have to think about in this body, eliminating the Select Committee on Narcotics, I just think that it was a decision that we should not have made.

And I am hoping that as a result of it, you don't give up the fight, that you continue to fight even though for some reason, this body felt that the committee should not continue.

So thank you very much, Congressman Rangel, for all you do.

Mr. RANGEL. Thank you.

And I thank all the members of the committee.

Mr. TOWNS. Thank you very much.

Let me say at this time that there is a vote on the floor, and what I would suggest is that we just break and go over. And I hope that all the Members will return as soon as they vote, come right back so that we can continue with our next witness.

It is a temporary recess.

[Recess taken.]

Mr. TOWNS. We will reconvene.

At this time, let me call on our second witness. It is Dr. Dan Melnick, Director of the Office of Applied Statistics for the Substance Abuse and Mental Health Services Administration.

Dr. Melnick, we look forward to hearing from you. We understand that you spent a lot of years here on the Hill, so we are interested in hearing from you and in the administration's findings relating to increased drug use.

STATEMENT OF DANIEL MELNICK, Ph.D., ACTING DEPUTY DIRECTOR, OFFICE OF APPLIED STUDIES, SUBSTANCE ABUSE AND MENTAL HEALTH SERVICES ADMINISTRATION, U.S. DEPARTMENT OF HEALTH AND HUMAN SERVICES

Dr. MELNICK. Good morning. I am Acting Deputy Director of the Office Applied Studies in the Substance Abuse and Mental Health

Services Administration, SAMHSA. I am very pleased to be here and to report to you on the results of our DAWN study.

First of all, I would like to request that my full statement and our April 1993 quarterly advanced report on this topic and several charts and tables be included in the record.

Mr. TOWNS. Without objection.

Dr. MELNICK. This morning I am going to concentrate on some main points. My testimony is based on the recent results from SAMHSA's Drug Abuse Warning Network [DAWN] survey tracking a number of drug-related emergency room episodes based on a sample of hospitals from around the Nation. These episodes are identified by hospital staff when drug abuse is implicated in causing a problem.

A cadre of reporters identified cases in which a person's health problem resulted from the effects of drug abuse and they ended up in the emergency room. They do this based on the review of emergency room nurses and physician's notes. These are people that work in the hospital, so they are intimately familiar with the conditions and can do the best job of interpreting the data.

We depend on the cooperation of the emergency room staff in carefully recording these conditions, and we are very grateful to the hospitals for their participation.

Actually, Mr. Chairman, we take extraordinary care to protect the identity of the cooperating hospitals, staff, and patients who are doing this for us. In fact, our files never contained names or identifying information of patients because we believe they should be protected.

The DAWN results do not provide a complete picture of drug abuse problems. It is important to recognize that. But rather, they focus on the impact that these problems have on our Nations's emergency rooms. If a person is admitted to another part of the hospital for treatment or if they are treated in a doctor's office or at a treatment center, DAWN would not include the episode.

DAWN covers episodes resulting from a patient's own drug abuse problem. We do not include cases in which another person's drug abuse led to an event which caused the person's problem.

For example, if a driver is in an accident and they end up in the emergency room and it is determined that the accident occurred because they were impaired due to drug abuse, we will include them in our reports. But if the same person happened to be sitting in the passenger seat of the car and they were impaired due to drug abuse, we don't include them because the drug abuse did not directly contribute to their problem.

We do this because we have discovered over the years that if we don't have this kind of limitation, we will have a great deal of difficulty interpreting the physicians' and nurses' notes on which this survey is based. It means that DAWN only provides an indication of the problem. It by no means tells us about the total number of cases in the emergency room which can be traced to drug abuse.

Nevertheless, we think it provides important and useful data.

What I would like to do next is to talk about some of the results from our most recent report. What we have done here is to reanalyze the results for you so you can see trends over longer periods of time than were actually contained in the advance report.

In the first three-quarters of 1992, taken as a whole, we found that drug-related emergency room visits, all of them taken together for the Nation, increased by 7 percent over the similar period, the first three-quarters of 1991, that is January to September in both years.

About 320,000 out of 63 million emergency room visits in the Nation were wholly or partly caused by drug abuse. About 125,000 of these were cases in which somebody had tried to commit suicide, and about 128,000 involved drug dependence or use for psychic effects. There were a large number that the hospital was simply unable to determine the reason why the drugs were being used, so we included them in our statistics but couldn't break it out this way. Just under 40,000 cases involved people who were seeking help in overcoming their drug-related problems through detoxification or the management of withdrawal.

DAWN cases are concentrated in the inner cities. From January to September 1992, more than half of all the episodes, or about 170,000 episodes, occurred in 21 metropolitan areas for which we collect separate statistics. Sixteen of these areas reported increases in that period of time.

The first chart, over here—there are copies also in your packet—shows the number of drug abuse episodes in a selected set of cities. There are two bars for each city. The top one shows the number in the first 9 months of 1991, and the bottom one shows a similar number for the first 9 months of 1992.

In the New York metropolitan area 31,000 drug episodes occurred making it the largest center for these problems in the Nation, followed by Los Angeles, Philadelphia, Detroit, and Chicago.

New York had the largest absolute increase in the number of drug-related cases. It also included proportionately fewer suicides, meaning that we were reporting more drug abuse cases due to causes, other than suicides.

Of course, the number of cases varies with the size of the population of these places. If you have more people in a place, you will have more cases just because of that. And to control for population size, we calculated the chance that a visit to an emergency room would involve drugs compared to the average visit in the Nation. The results are presented in chart 2.

Now, the top line of this chart, the one at the very top, represents the national average. And we have set it to 1 so that you could easily see the comparisons while the lines for each metropolitan area show their relative position, relative to the national average. We have shown three lines for each area: the whole metropolitan area, the central city, and the rest of the area. You can see that there is really quite a bit of difference among the metropolitan areas. Generally, the central cities have much higher relative rates of drug abuse related cases in the emergency rooms.

In the central cities of the 21 DAWN metropolitan areas, taken together as a whole for all these areas, an emergency room visit is actually 2.6 times as likely to involve drugs as the national average visit. While the visit in an area outside of the central cities is only a third, that is 0.32 percent likely to involve drugs.

In no case is one of these metropolitan areas less than the national average. In San Francisco, Detroit, Newark, Baltimore, and

Philadelphia, the central city rates are more than 3 times the national average. And the central city in New York—and that is New York City—is 2.9 times the national average, showing how these cases are really very much concentrated. And there is a greater impact in the central city emergency rooms than there is outside of them.

Our data also make it possible to focus on cases which involve specific drugs. And today we are going to talk about heroin and cocaine. We examined trends and episodes involving heroin and cocaine. Chart 3 shows that in the period since 1988, reported emergency room episodes remained relatively stable.

The red line on this chart shows the total number of episodes for all reasons, while the yellow line shows the cocaine episodes, and the blue dotted line shows the heroin episodes.

However, if we compare the first three-quarters of 1991 to the first three-quarters of 1992, which is a much shorter period of time going back to 1988, we find that heroin-related visits increased from 28,000 in the first 9-month period, to 35,000 in the 9-month period in 1991, or a 25 percent increase. While cocaine-related visits increased from 76,000 to 88,000 or about 16 percent increase.

We have also seen a shift in the age composition of people showing up in emergency rooms for drug-related problems. Since 1988, the proportion of heroin or cocaine-related episodes that involve people 26 years or older increased.

Chart 4 shows the heroin trends for age groups. The red line shows the number of episodes involving people over age 35. The yellow line shows those age 26 to 34, while the blue line shows those age 18 to 25.

Between the first three-quarters of 1991, and the same period in 1992, there was a 36 percent increase among those aged over 35 and older and a 12 percent increase among those age 26 to 34.

Chart 5 shows the same trends for cocaine. Between the first three-quarters of 1991 and 1992, there was a 34 percent increase in cocaine-related episodes among those age 35 and older and an 11 percent increase among those age 26 to 34.

In the central cities of the 21 metropolitan areas that we tracked, in this same time period, there was an increase of 25 percent in heroin-related emergency room episodes and an increase of 20 percent in cocaine-related episodes.

Chart 6 shows that there is considerable variation in the heroin trends among metropolitan areas. And we have just given some examples. Since 1990, Baltimore and New York have both experienced large increases in the number of heroin cases appearing in emergency room. But Los Angeles and Newark, for example, have only experienced small increases or hardly any increases at all. In this period, the number of heroin cases in New York more than doubled from about 1,000 each quarter to more than 2,200. Baltimore increased from less than 500 in the first quarter of 1990 to almost 1,500 in the third quarter of 1992.

Chart 7 shows the same trends for cocaine. Here, too, there is wide variation in the trends. Since 1990, New York increased from slightly more than 3,000 cocaine cases per quarter to more than 5,000 in the third quarter of 1992. Baltimore went from less than

1,000 cases in the first quarter of 1990 to more than 2,000 in the third quarter of 1992.

At the same time, Los Angeles and Newark report little change.

Mr. Chairman, our testimony has illustrated the impact that drug abuse has on hospital emergency rooms. It has shown how this is a particularly important problem for central cities.

I would be very happy to answer any questions relating to the survey and its results.

[The prepared statement of Dr. Melnick follows:]

Testimony of
Daniel Melnick, Ph.D.
Acting Deputy Director
Office of Applied Studies
Substance Abuse and
Mental Health Services Administration

Before the
House Government Operations
Committee

Subcommittee on Human Resources
Intergovernmental Relations

May 26, 1993

SAMHSA SUBSTANCE ABUSE AND MENTAL HEALTH SERVICES ADMINISTRATION
U.S. Department of Health and Human Services
Public Health Service

Mr. Chairman. I am Daniel Melnick, Acting Deputy director of the Office of Applied Studies, in the Substance Abuse and Mental Health Services Administration [SAMHSA] . I am pleased to have this opportunity to discuss the impact of drug abuse problems on hospital emergency rooms. I am submitting a copy of our most recent advance report on this topic and ask that it be included in the record of this hearing.

The DAWN Survey

Since the early 1970's, the Drug Abuse Warning Network [DAWN] has tracked the number of drug related emergency room episodes based on a sample of hospitals from around the Nation. These episodes are identified by hospital staff when drug abuse is implicated in causing the problem.

The DAWN survey was started in the Drug Enforcement Administration and transferred to the National Institute on Drug Abuse in 1980. In 1988, NIDA fully implemented a new sampling procedure that makes it possible to produce national estimates as well as those for 21 major metropolitan areas. SAMHSA was given responsibility for this project as a result of the ADAMHA Reorganization Act which took effect on October 1, 1992.

The DAWN results provide a running account of the identified impact of drug abuse on the emergency departments of the Nation's hospitals. It is based on a sample of non-federal short stay general hospitals in the United States excluding Alaska and Hawaii. We

rely on a cadre of trained reporters [one in each sampled hospital] who help us to identify cases in which a person's health problem resulted from the effects of drug abuse. These reporters are nurses or other medical personnel who review hospital charts in the sampled emergency rooms for indications -- noted by physicians and nurses who treated the patients -- that drug abuse was a cause of the visit to the emergency room. Thus, the accuracy of these reports depends critically on the cooperation of the emergency room staff in carefully recording these conditions. SAMHSA compensates the hospitals for these efforts by their staff.

Privacy Protection

Mr. Chairman. We take extraordinary care to protect the identity of the cooperating hospitals, staff and patients. In fact, our files never contain the names or identifying information of patients.

Limits of the Data

It is important to recognize that the DAWN results do not provide a complete picture of drug abuse problems, but rather focus on the impact that these problems have on our Nation's emergency rooms. If a person is admitted to another part of the hospital for treatment, treated in a physician's office or at a treatment center, DAWN would not include the episode.

DAWN covers episodes resulting from the patient's own drug abuse. We do not include cases in which another person's drug abuse led to an event which caused the patient's problem. Thus, when drivers are involved in an accident while they are impaired

because of drug use, we report the episodes in DAWN. But, when passengers are injured and they or the drivers are impaired because of drug abuse, we do not report the episodes.

Thus, DAWN only provides an indication of the problem. It by no means tells us about its total magnitude--nor does it tell us about the total number of cases in the emergency room which can be traced to drug abuse. It does provide a consistent measure that has been collected for several years. We can use it to report on the trends in drug related emergency room episodes and the places where this problem is concentrated. This means that the changes in DAWN -- the trends and the reports of "hot spots" -- are probably more indicative than the actual magnitudes we report.

Latest Results

When we examined the reports from the Nation's hospitals for the first three quarters of 1992, we found:

* Drug-related emergency room visits increased by 7% over the first three quarters of 1991.

* About 320 thousand out of the 63 million emergency room visits in the Nation were wholly or partly caused by drug abuse.

* About 125 thousand of the drug related episodes were attempted suicides, while about 128 thousand involved drug dependence or casual use. [The hospitals were not able to report the reason for the abuse in the remainder of the cases.]

* Just under 40 thousand cases involved people who were seeking help in overcoming their drug related problems through detoxification or the management of withdrawal.

DAWN Cases Are Concentrated in the Inner Cities

Mr. Chairman. We analyzed the DAWN data to locate the places where the emergency rooms are more impacted by the drug problem. More than half of all the episodes or about 170 thousand occurred in the 21 metropolitan areas for which we collect separate statistics. There were a total of about 17 million emergency room visits in these metropolitan areas. Increases in drug related emergency room episodes were seen in 16 of those metropolitan areas.

We also calculated the chance that a visit to an emergency room would involve drugs compared to the average visit in the total United States.

* In the 21 DAWN metropolitan areas taken as a whole, an emergency room visit in a central city is 2.6 times as likely to involve drugs as the national average; while a visit in an area outside the central cities is only 0.32 times as likely to involve drugs.

* Here are some examples of the relative probabilities for central cities:

- San Francisco	5.6
- Detroit	3.8
- Baltimore	3.6
- Newark	3.7
- Philadelphia	3.6
- New York City	2.9
- Miami	2.7
- Seattle	2.4

- Los Angeles 2.2

Of course, the actual number of cases also varies with the size of the population in these places. 33 thousand of the DAWN episodes occurred in the New York Metropolitan area making it the largest center of drug related emergency room episodes in the Nation, followed by Los Angeles, Philadelphia, Chicago, and Detroit. New York had the largest absolute increase in the number of drug related cases between 1991 and 1992. Cases reported in New York also tend to include proportionally fewer suicides.

HEROIN AND COCAINE

Our data make it possible to focus on cases which involve specific drugs. We examined trends in episodes involving heroin and cocaine. In the period since 1988, reported emergency room episodes involving heroin and cocaine have remained relatively stable for the Nation. However, if we compare the first 3 quarters of 1991 to the first 3 quarters of 1992, we find that Heroin-related visits increased from 28,000 to 34,900, an increase of 25%, while Cocaine-related visits increased 16% from 75,900 to 87,900.

We have seen a shift in the age composition of people showing up in emergency rooms for drug related problems. Since 1988, the proportion of heroin or cocaine related episodes that involved people who were 26 years or older increased.

Specifically, with regard to Heroin,

- **Between the first 3 quarters of 1991 and the first 3 quarters of 1992, there was a 36% increase among those aged 35 and older and a 12% increase among those aged 26-34.**

- **There was an increase of 25% among those living in the 21 DAWN central cities of the metropolitan areas.**

- **There was an increase of 39% among men and no change among women.**

- **The main motive given for heroin use in emergency room patients was dependence and the number citing dependence rose by 21%.**

- **The main reasons reported for the heroin-related visits were overdose and chronic effects. Overdose cases rose by 57% and chronic effects episodes by 24%.**

With regard to cocaine;

- **There was a 34% increase among those aged 35 and older and a 11% increase among those aged 26-34.**

- **20% among those living in the central cities of the 21 DAWN metropolitan areas.**

- There was an increase of 19% among men and 9% among women.

- The main motive given for cocaine use was dependence and the number citing dependence rose by 16%.

- The main reasons reported for the cocaine-related visits were seeking detoxification and an unexpected reaction. Seeking detoxification rose by 17% and unexpected reaction rose by 16%.

We also traced the changes in recent years in some of the metropolitan areas for which we have data:

* Since 1990, Baltimore and New York have both experienced large increases in the number of heroin cases showing up in emergency rooms. In this period, the number of heroin cases in New York more than doubled from about 1000 in each quarter to more than 2200. Baltimore increased from less than 500 per quarter in 1990 to almost 1500 in the third quarter of 1992.

* Since 1990, New York hospitals report an increase from slightly more than 3000 cocaine cases per quarter to more than 5000 cases in the third quarter of 1992. There were similar increases in Baltimore from less than 1000 per quarter in 1990 to more than 2000 in the third quarter of 1992.

Mr. Chairman. Our testimony has illustrated the impact that drug abuse has on hospital emergency rooms. It has shown how this is a particularly important problem for central cities. I would be happy to answer any questions you may have.

Number of Drug-Related Emergency Room Visits

For Selected Metropolitan Areas,

1st 3 Quarters 1991 and 1st 3 Quarters 1992

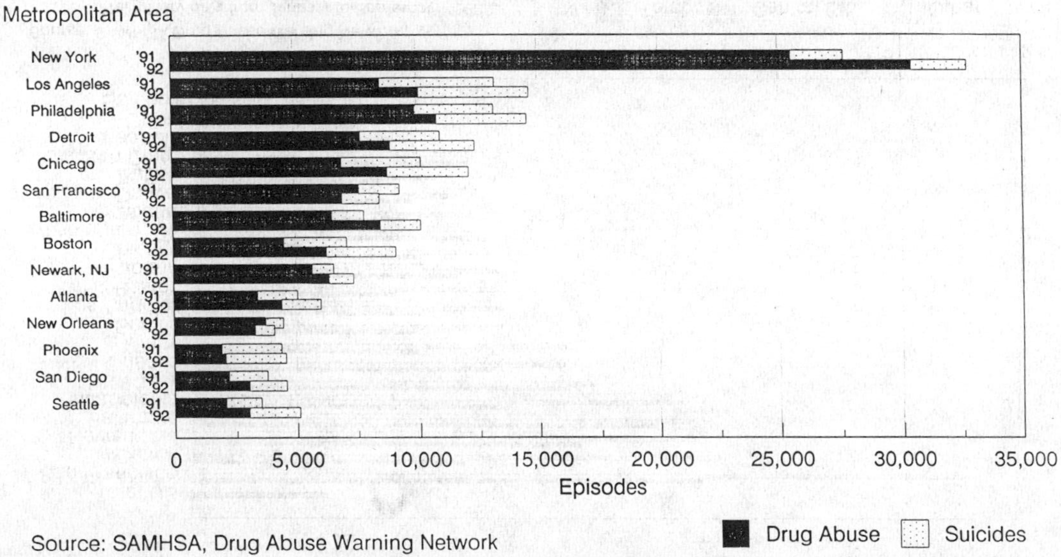

Source: SAMHSA, Drug Abuse Warning Network

SAMHSA SUBSTANCE ABUSE AND MENTAL HEALTH SERVICES ADMINISTRATION
U.S. Department of Health and Human Services
Public Health Service

Comparative Risk of ai. Emergency Room Visit
Involving Drug Abuse
Selected Metropolitan Areas Compared with the US Average

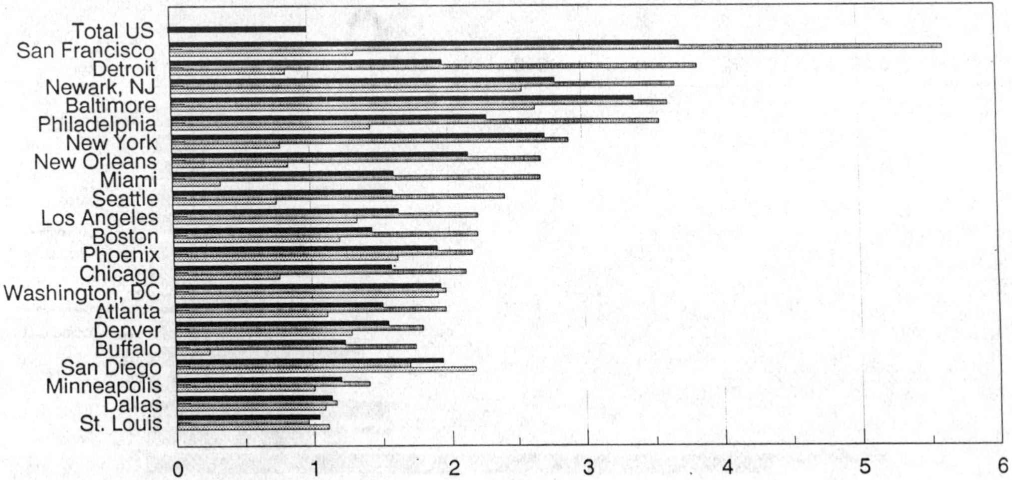

Source: SAMHSA Drug Abuse Warning Network;
Preliminary data from January to September 1992

SAMHSA SUBSTANCE ABUSE AND MENTAL HEALTH SERVICES ADMINISTRATION
U.S. Department of Health and Human Services
Public Health Service

Trends in Drug-Related Emergencies

Total Episodes, Cocaine and Heroin Mentions by Quarter, 1988 - 1992

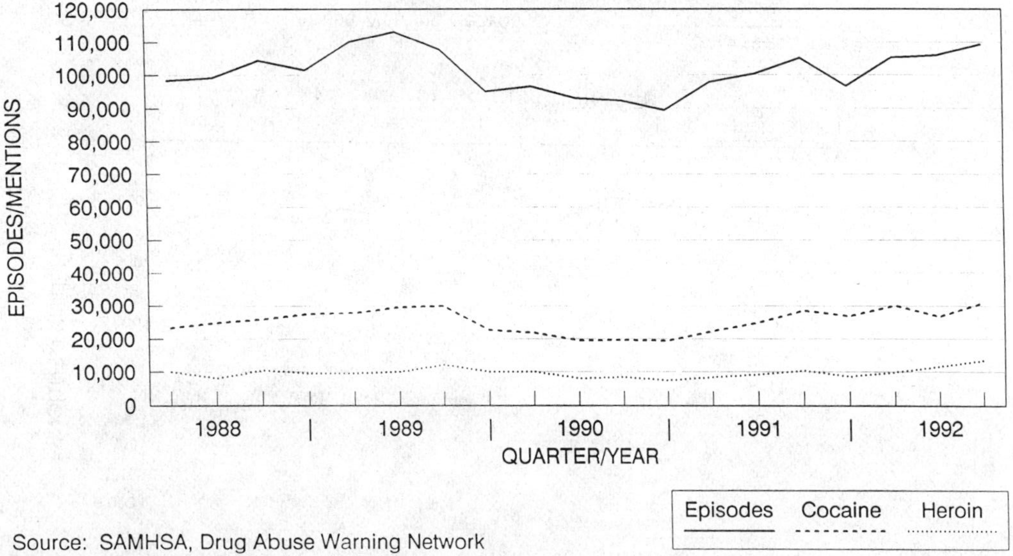

Source: SAMHSA, Drug Abuse Warning Network

SAMHSA SUBSTANCE ABUSE AND MENTAL HEALTH SERVICES ADMINISTRATION
U.S. Department of Health and Human Services
Public Health Service

Trends in Heroin-Related Emergencies

Quarterly Heroin Mentions by Age, 1988-1992

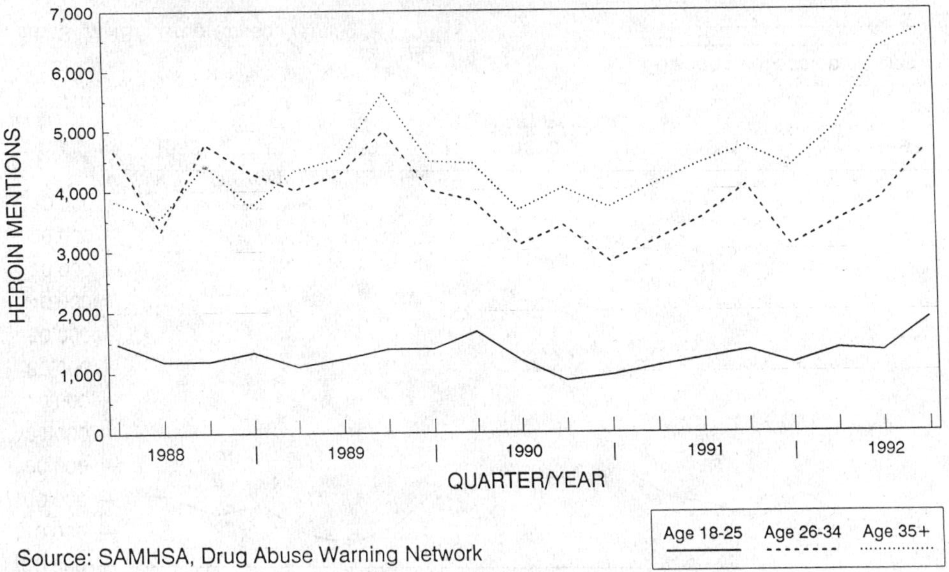

Source: SAMHSA, Drug Abuse Warning Network

SAMHSA SUBSTANCE ABUSE AND MENTAL HEALTH SERVICES ADMINISTRATION
U.S. Department of Health and Human Services
Public Health Service

Trends in Drug-Related Emergencies

Quarterly Cocaine Mentions by Age, 1988-1992

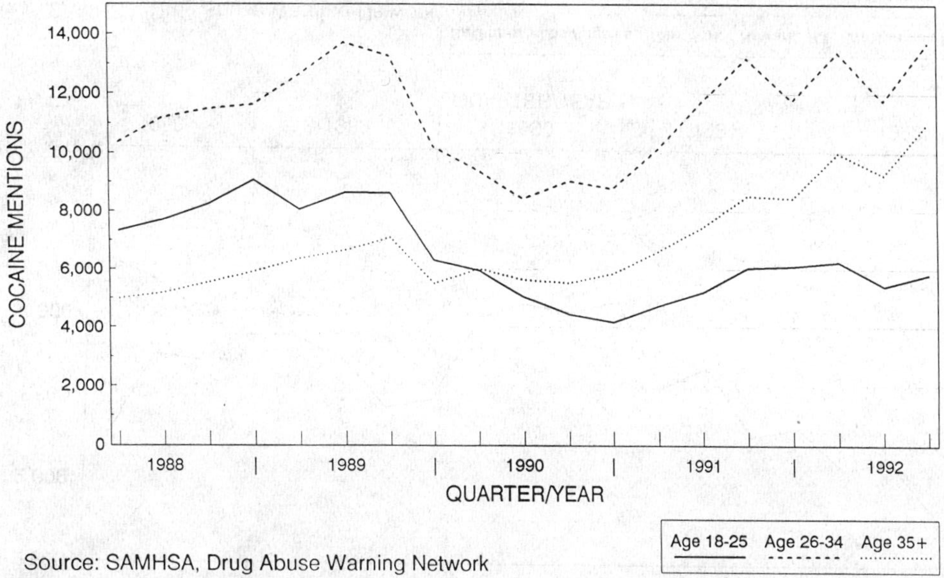

Source: SAMHSA, Drug Abuse Warning Network

SAMHSA SUBSTANCE ABUSE AND MENTAL HEALTH SERVICES ADMINISTRATION
U.S. Department of Health and Human Services
Public Health Service

Trends in Heroin-Related Emergency Room
Episodes for Selected Metropolitan Areas, by Quarter, 1988 - 1992

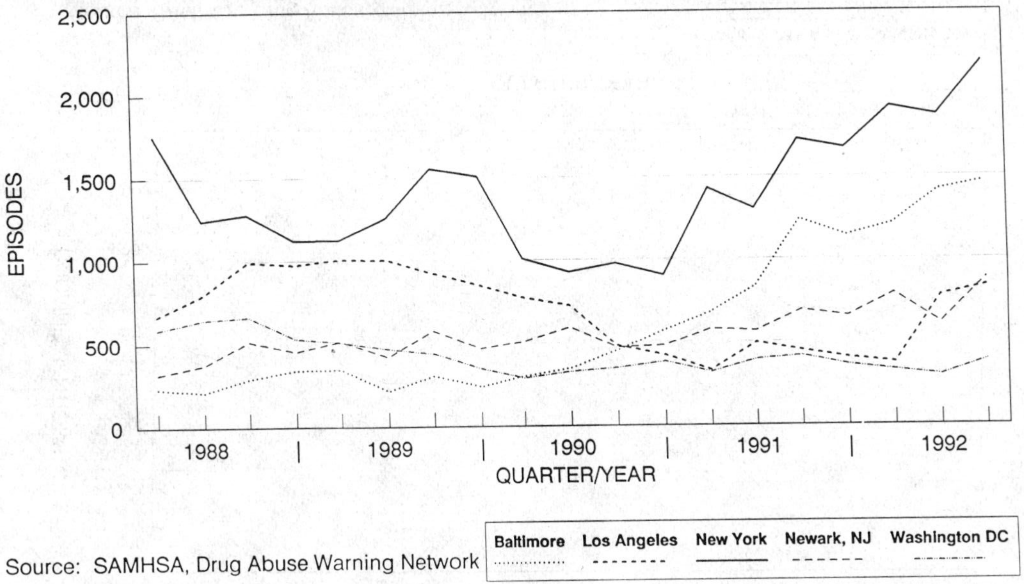

Source: SAMHSA, Drug Abuse Warning Network

SAMHSA SUBSTANCE ABUSE AND MENTAL HEALTH SERVICES ADMINISTRATION
U.S. Department of Health and Human Services
Public Health Service

Trends in Cocaine-Related Emergency Room Episodes for Selected Metropolitan Areas, by Quarter, 1988 - 1992

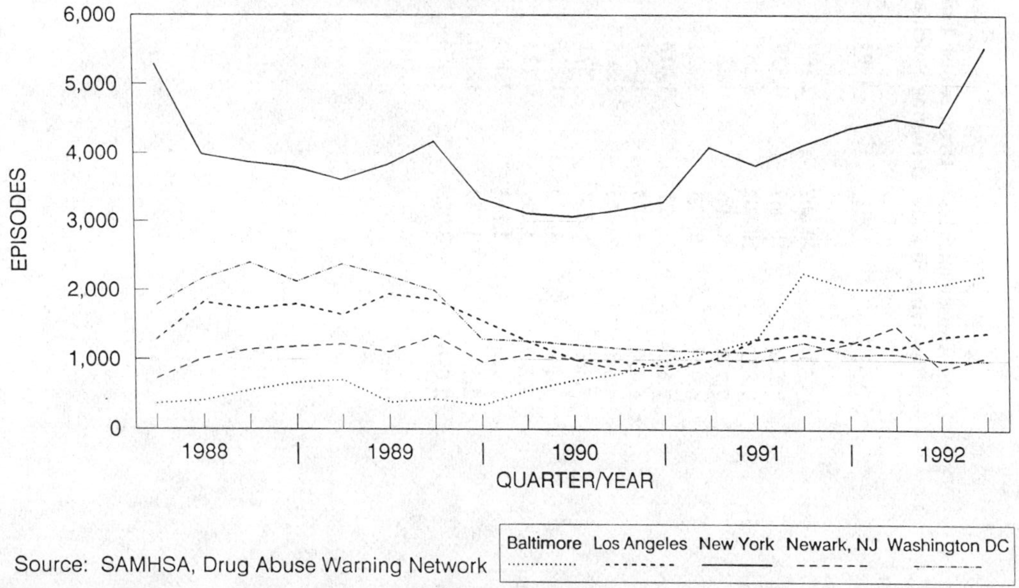

Source: SAMHSA, Drug Abuse Warning Network

SAMHSA SUBSTANCE ABUSE AND MENTAL HEALTH SERVICES ADMINISTRATION
U.S. Department of Health and Human Services
Public Health Service

Number of Drug-Related Emergency Room Visits For Selected Metropolitan Areas First 3 Quarters 1991 and First 3 Quarters 1992

Metropolitan Area	Drug Abuse Episodes Not Involving Suicide		Drug Abuse Episodes Involving Suicide	
	1991	1992	1991	1992
New York	25,534	30,407	2,107	2,309
Los Angeles	8,552	10,067	4,679	4,549
Philadelphia	9,891	10,802	3,284	3,721
Detroit	7,730	8,896	3,232	3,474
Chicago	6,928	8,773	3,221	3,339
San Francisco	7,655	6,927	1,618	1,514
Baltimore	6,497	8,473	1,337	1,622
Boston	4,546	6,243	2,565	2,819
Newark, NJ	5,680	6,334	871	1,017
Atlanta	3,440	4,423	1,626	1,582
New Orleans	3,722	3,299	722	786
Phoenix	1,926	2,113	2,469	2,479
San Diego	2,230	3,039	1,570	1,531
Seattle	2,090	3,025	1,454	2,058

Comparative Risk of An Emergency Room Visit Involving Drugs Abuse
Selected Metropolitan Areas Compared with the US Average

	Total	Central City	Other
Total US	1.00		
Atlanta	1.51	1.964	1.106
Baltimore	3.38	3.620	2.660
Boston	1.44	2.215	1.206
Buffalo	1.23	1.747	0.252
Chicago	1.58	2.120	0.765
Dallas	1.13	1.162	1.082
Denver	1.55	1.801	1.279
Detroit	1.97	3.843	0.833
Los Angeles	1.64	2.218	1.333
Miami	1.61	2.693	0.351
Minneapolis	1.20	1.402	1.009
New Orleans	2.15	2.698	0.842
New York	2.73	2.903	0.785
Newark	2.81	3.678	2.568
Philadelphia	2.30	3.557	1.440
Phoenix	1.91	2.170	1.630
St. Louis	1.04	0.961	1.105
San Diego	1.94	1.705	2.178
San Francisco	3.72	5.620	1.330
Seattle	1.60	2.429	0.752
District Columbia	1.93	1.968	1.909

Trends in Drug-Related Emergencies
Total Episodes, Cocaine and Heroin Mentions
by Quarter, 1988 - 1992

Year	Quarter	Episodes	Cocaine	Heroin
1988	1	98,415	23,366	10,014
	2	99,224	24,857	8,097
	3	104,432	25,855	10,463
	4	101,507	27,501	9,489
1989	1	110,111	27,803	9,550
	2	113,141	29,625	10,050
	3	94,994	22,646	9,960
	4	96,545	21,853	9,967
1990	1	93,010	19,453	8,059
	2	92,328	19,668	3,348
	3	89,325	19,381	7,510
	4	97,858	22,330	8,387
1991	1	100,396	24,970	9,228
	2	105,147	28,552	10,338
	3	96,678	26,875	8,623
	4	105,378	30,103	9,947
1992	1	106,024	26,854	11,581
	2	109,241	30,924	13,387

Trends in Drug-Related Emergencies
Quarterly Heroin Mentions by Age, 1988-1992

Year	Quarter	Age 18 - 25	26 - 34	35+
1988	1	1,478	4,655	3,828
	2	1,186	3,329	3,545
	3	1,186	4,774	4,426
	4	1,336	4,303	3,735
1989	1	1,224	4,264	4,525
	2	1,383	4,982	5,615
	3	1,386	3,993	4,475
	4	1,668	3,826	4,447
1990	1	1,189	3,088	3,670
	2	857	3,407	4,027
	3	941	2,805	3,707
	4	1,087	3,158	4,095
1991	1	1,227	3,523	4,431
	2	1,354	4,066	4,724
	3	1,134	3,066	4,381
	4	1,369	3,460	5,014
1992	1	1,324	3,844	6,348
	2	1,869	4,680	6,693

Trends in Drug-Related Emergeencies
Quarterly Cocaine Mentions by Age, 1988-1992

		Age		
Year	Quarter	18 - 25	26 - 34	35+
1988	1	7,318	10,363	4,977
	2	7,699	11,184	5,188
	3	8,240	11,472	5,554
	4	9,065	11,184	5,188
1989	1	8,052	12,626	6,367
	2	8,621	13,712	6,661
	3	8,611	13,262	7,087
	4	6,316	10,218	5,512
1990	1	5,957	9,388	6,032
	2	5,042	8,440	5,635
	3	4,440	9,039	5,530
	4	4.175	8,772	5,857
1991	1	4,740	10,146	6,629
	2	5,042	8,440	5,635
	3	4,440	9,039	5,530
	4	4,175	8,772	5,857
1992	1	6,245	13,393	9,994
	2	5,411	11,770	9,252
	3	5,812	13,703	11,019

Trends in Heroin-Related Emergency Room Episodes for Selected Metropolitan Areas, by Quarter, 1988-1992

Year, Quarter		Baltimore	Los Angeles	New York	Newark	Washington
1988	1	229	670	1,755	315	587
	2	207	798	1,240	373	648
	3	288	992	1,279	516	665
	4	338	973	1,120	451	533
1989	1	341	1,005	1,123	516	511
	2	212	1,003	1,254	419	468
	3	300	924	1,553	576	437
	4	235	848	1,507	467	345
1990	1	298	773	1,005	508	287
	2	343	726	925	595	322
	3	451	482	976	470	345
	4	575	422	904	481	381
1991	1	681	327	1,429	581	316
	2	836	495	1,301	570	392
	3	1,235	447	1,722	692	413
	4	1,139	403	1,671	658	359
1992	1	1,211	373	1,919	793	325
	2	1,416	779	1,867	616	295
	3	1,469	837	2,191	883	386

Trends in Cocaine-Related Emergency Room Episodes for Selected Metropolitan Areas, by Quarter, 1988-1992

Year, Quarter		Baltimore	Los Angeles	New York	Newark	Washington
1988	1	366	1,290	5,284	728	1,783
	2	410	1,822	3,983	1,016	2,176
	3	552	1,728	3,863	1,144	2,397
	4	666	1,799	3,786	1,182	2,123
1989	1	696	1,643	3,602	1,215	2,377
	2	380	1,939	3,826	1,102	2,202
	3	425	1,860	4,171	1,341	1,984
	4	339	1,557	3,326	960	1,291
1990	1	547	1,259	3,109	1,066	1,266
	2	700	997	3,069	994	1,217
	3	791	970	3,169	842	1,164
	4	986	903	3,286	851	1,141
1991	1	1,112	985	4,084	995	1,123
	2	1,304	1,297	3,819	974	1,112
	3	2,248	1,361	4,112	1,110	1,252
	4	2,023	1,255	4,362	1,239	1,084
1992	1	2,013	1,169	4,505	1,482	1,088
	2	2,093	1,338	4,398	872	990
	3	2,226	1,394	5,535	1,049	996

Mr. TOWNS. Thank you very much, Dr. Melnick. I would like to ask one question, and then I am going to yield to the ranking person on the subcommittee.

Why do you think that the older addict is having more problems than the younger addict? I thought it would be the other way around.

Dr. MELNICK. Well, Mr. Chairman, first of all, you have to understand that the survey is a survey of episodes. That is to say, our unit of measure is a person showing up in an emergency room who is identified as having a drug problem and that drug problem caused the reason why they were there.

Unfortunately, the same person may show up more than once in our statistics, unfortunately for that person. A person who is older may tend to have more problems that cause a medical emergency that bring them into the emergency room. That is one possible reason.

Another possible reason is that there is a cohort of people who started into drug abuse sometime ago, and they are now coming into this age group. And we believe from other work that we are doing that this is a good part of the explanation.

There is, in these numbers, one encouraging thing to report. And that is the relative stability or almost slight declines among those people who are in younger groups because, hopefully, that means that later on that will carry forward to other reductions.

Suffice it to say that, there are these two possible explanations, or some combination of them; and we don't know the full answer. But we think this is a part of the explanation.

Mr. TOWNS. Thank you very much.

Congressman Schiff.

Mr. SCHIFF. Thank you, Mr. Chairman.

I just want to say that I appreciated Dr. Melnick—your presentation. I think that you were very articulate in what you told us about. And I followed your graphs, and I have no questions. That is not disinterest. I think I got the message. Thank you.

Mr. TOWNS. Thank you, Congressman Payne.

Mr. PAYNE. Yes.

Let me ask you in your statistics, have you determined that there is an increase in heroin use over cocaine in the past 2 to 3 years?

Dr. MELNICK. What this survey tells us, Congressman, is that the number of people showing up in the emergency room with a problem has increased. It is a survey that is really intended to tell us more about the emergency room than it is about the people. It shows the pressures that occur in the emergency room due to heroin and cocaine.

But one of the limitations of the survey is that it cannot tell us—unfortunately this one can't; however, we do other surveys—about what is happening in the general population. There may be some people—and one of the reasons why the statistics for DAWN show greater numbers in the central cities is certainly because they are there, but it is also because people outside the central cities may be using other parts of the medical system when they have problems like this. And so they simply don't show up.

But to conclude, from this survey itself we cannot say anything very much about the overall—what is happening in the population with regard to drug problems. We can just talk about the hospitals.

Mr. PAYNE. With the whole question of health care reform, have you been involved in the—or has your office been involved in the whole discussion that Mrs. Hillary Rodham Clinton is having as relates to this situation?

Dr. MELNICK. I think it is fair to say, since it appeared in the Wall Street Journal and the New York Times, that I and two other members of my staff were involved as members, worker bees, in that project. And we provided them with a lot of data.

Mr. PAYNE. Being from Newark and seeing the statistics of which I am currently aware, I think Congressman Rangel was talking about the need to have some alternatives to curb the large number of drug sales that occur which, therefore, result in a high incidence of substance abuse.

Have you made any recommendations on what you consider would be a moving toward a solution to the problem?

Dr. MELNICK. Our office really has the role of providing the numbers, the statistics that relate to these problems and doing it in a straightforward way for all consumers, for you, for the task force, or anyone else who asks. And we are not the right people to be in the business of making direct recommendations in regard to that. We have certainly shared our information widely, and we will continue to do it.

Mr. PAYNE. Just a last question. Generally, in the inner cities where poor people or minority people live, statistics are much more readily available. I mean, you know, I was born in Newark and lived there all my life and still live there and intend to stay there. So, I guess, I have been counted in about a hundred different statistics. We are always counted. Minorities are statistics prone.

The suburban communities don't tend to be under that much scrutiny. It seems that the statistics—people are not as statistically vulnerable as in inner cities. Have you done suburban communities? Do you do cities in general? And do you feel that the reporting in other places is as accurate as in inner cities?

For example, in suburban communities, a person who may be picked up for drunk driving is driven home by the policeman because he is the local banker and they say, you know, you probably had one too many, Mr. Jones; here is your key; don't do it again, you might get somebody injured. And that is good, because the main thing is getting someone off the road and keeping the incident off the record.

Of course, if you were in downtown Newark and you were wavering and you are pulled over and several cops have their guns pulled and you are locked up for DWI, which should be, too, it goes on the record.

My question, I guess, is—and even incidents of drug abuse in suburban communities in schools tend not to be, from what I have been told—or let me say the rumor has it that they are not reported as concisely as the statistically concentrated areas like inner cities.

Do you feel that this is just an erroneous assumption? Or do you believe there is some validity in my notion?

Dr. MELNICK. I think you have asked a very important question here. And I want to thank you for it because it gives me an opportunity to talk not only about this survey but some of the other work that we are doing.

First of all, the first thing to say about the DAWN survey on which we have reported is that it is constructed as a sample to represent the whole of the United States, and all kinds of places are included in it. It is not merely focused in the central cities.

In fact, in the material I have presented here, we have shown the difference between the results that we get in the central city and the results that we get outside of the central city. We have not just reported on the central city.

The second chart that we used, for example, clearly showed the differences between the two. The second thing to say about it is that, however, the design of this survey—and it has been going now since the early 1970's—is based on the assumption that what is important to measure is the interaction between people who have problems with substance abuse and emergency rooms. So it is a limited effort focused on that.

I would contend it is an important effort because we need to know the effect that these problems are having on the emergency rooms. But in my prepared testimony, I was quite candid with you to say that we don't believe that this describes the whole problem. There probably needs to be other indicators, and SAMHSA being a relatively young agency, only having started in October—and as the Congressman mentioned, I had a long career prior to that and just came into this work recently—we are certainly going to be looking at ways of improving the statistical work that we do in order to provide broader coverage.

And I should probably add that SAMHSA, as an agency, has started support programs and will continue to support programs to strengthen the State capacities to collect better data for all kinds of areas within their State.

I know, for example, that a study done in the State of South Carolina which involved taking toxicological tests of women giving birth, actually found quite high rates, as high or sometimes higher rates of women who gave birth to children and who were obviously affected by cocaine abuse in some of the rural areas of South Carolina as they found in some of the city areas of that State.

So certainly this is an issue, and it is an important one, and it is one that we think needs some attention. I should also mention, of course, that we do other studies. We do a household survey on drug abuse. And in that study, we report in detail on the differences in substance abuse in different areas of the country, different types of places. And there, because we are doing household interviews, we have coverage that isn't impacted by the fact that we are going to emergency rooms.

Mr. PAYNE. Thank you very much.

Mr. TOWNS. Thank you.

We have been joined by Congressman Craig Washington, of Houston, TX. I yield to him at this time for any questions or comments that he might have.

Mr. WASHINGTON. Thank you. I apologize to you and the other witnesses for my tardiness. Unfortunately, I had two subcommittees meeting at the same time. I am on the Committee on Energy and Commerce's Subcommittee on Energy and Power.

I did, however, Dr. Melnick, overnight have an opportunity to read your testimony in its entirety as well as its preliminary estimates from the Drug Abuse Warning Network advance report.

And I would like to thank the chairman and ranking member for holding this important hearing and Congressman Rangel who has previously testified for the important testimony that you gave on this body of knowledge.

If I may, I have just several questions. Let me start with a preparatory question please. And I apologize to you. I am new to the committee and also to the subcommittee, and I do not know your background.

What is your advanced degree in, please, sir?

Dr. MELNICK. I am a social scientist. I have a Ph.D. in social science. More precisely, political science. And after that, I worked for a number of years, 15 years at the Congressional Research Service in the Library of Congress where I served as the specialist in Federal Statistical Policy working on statistical issues that have to do with the government and the government's surveys.

At that time, I also did an awful lot of work related to the U.S. census and other related issues at the Bureau of Labor Statistics.

And I was an advisor to the House Post Office and Civil Service Committee in that role and served as an advisor to Chairman Hawkins on the Education, Labor Committee when he was doing work in the statistical area. For about 18 months I served as a technical staff member on detail from the Congressional Research Service to the staff of Chairman Sarbanes at the Joint Economic Committee working with them on the development of statistical work and surveys.

And then after that, I went back to the Congressional Research Service and subsequently went over to the National Science Foundation where I served as senior advisor for research methods in the Office of the Assistant Directorate of Education and Science, Education with Dr. Luther Williams.

And, subsequently, when SAMHSA was started last summer, Dr. Elaine Johnson, who is the Acting Administrator of SAMHSA, asked NSF if they would detail me over to work on the establishment of this new office because of my background in the area of statistical organizations.

Mr. WASHINGTON. So it can be truthfully said that you are an expert in the area of analysis?

Dr. MELNICK. I think so. And, I have access to a very fine staff of people with statistical backgrounds.

Mr. WASHINGTON. And I take that among the other things that you do is read from the publications of others in the area of statistical analysis?

Dr. MELNICK. I try to do as much of that as I can.

Mr. WASHINGTON. Now, then, that brings me, after that predicate, to several questions.

And then I will be finished, Mr. Chairman.

I read, as I said, with interest your testimony; and you elucidate very well on the focus that you brought here today and that the chairman requested and required of you with respect to the subject matter that brings us all together this morning.

One wonders if we could extrapolate from that, and I believe it would be within your purview; and if you feel comfortable giving an answer, I would appreciate it. And if you don't, say so, and I will understand.

I am a layperson in your field, attempting to define for myself a model by which I could be made to understand for the purpose of valid comparisons. I have not read or studied in your field. You are our expert in your field, so your opinion is important to me.

My question has to do with the opportunities that persons such as yourself have had or have undertaken having developed a statistical model, having reached a body of data with which you feel comfortable, and being able to report on the pattern that one develops within the area and the limited purview of our scope having to do with drug abuse.

And my question has to do with taking this model that you have made and the data that you have compiled, or others known to you by persons respected and known in the field, have you had an opportunity to make a comparison between the proportionate degree of change, if any, in certain locals, such as New York, Philadelphia, and the other cities that are mentioned, and compare those with the changes in the statute law with respect to the degree of severity of punishment for a person who is convicted of an offense for drug abuse.

Dr. MELNICK. We have not done that analysis. But I must say that I think your question is a very good one. I think it is very important for us to be taking data like this and relating it to the rest of the data and the rest of the information that we have.

As a matter of fact, one of the goals of the office is to do that. We have only been in operation now for a few months, but we have a prevalence branch, a group of analysts who have the assignment of trying to work with these data in combination with other data to try to make some more meaningful results from them.

Frankly, Congressman, we decided when we started this that we would have to try to do two things at the same time: We would have to try to address the very issues that you are raising with regard to improving our models at the same time that we continued to faithfully report the results from data that had been collected in the past. So that is where we are at right now.

We certainly think that is an important goal. We thank you for raising it. We share your concern, and we think it would be very important to do that.

Mr. WASHINGTON. Would you agree that, for policymakers such as ourselves, it would be helpful to us—let me put it that way—it would be helpful to us if we may know over the long course of history when we change the punishment for particular drug-related offenses, are we making a dent? Do we, in fact, decrease the amount of drug usage? Does it stay the same? Does it increase with respect to laws that become incrementally more severe with regard to persons—and I am not speaking of offenses related to the sale of drugs. I am speaking specifically to offenses related to the use of drugs.

Dr. MELNICK. I think it is a very important question that somebody should look at, and we certainly would be prepared to provide data to whichever analysts were doing it and to begin looking at it ourselves.

Mr. WASHINGTON. Thank you very much.

Thank you, Mr. Chairman.

Mr. TOWNS. Thank you very much. And I think your question was right on it. Earlier today Congressman Rangel talked about the $20 billion that we spend keeping young people in jail. And in New York it costs $60,000 a year to incarcerate someone.

So that question is really one that we need to know more about. We look at ways and methods to deal with it. We need to have as much information to deal with it. That is a key question.

Dr. MELNICK. Certainly the data that we have could be used that way, and we would be happy to help with it.

Mr. TOWNS. Thank you Dr. Melnick, for your testimony today. We appreciate your testimony. Thank you.

The next witnesses we will have are Dr. Elizabeth Sommers Strevey, senior vice president for the regulatory and professional affairs, Greater New York Hospital Association; and Dr. Beny Primm, executive director of the Addiction Research and Treatment Corp. of Brooklyn, NY.

If you could sum up your testimony in 5 minutes, your entire statement will be included in the record, if you would like. But if you would summarize, we would appreciate it.

Ms. Strevey, why don't you go first.

STATEMENT OF ELIZABETH SOMMERS STREVEY, SENIOR VICE PRESIDENT FOR REGULATORY AND PROFESSIONAL AFFAIRS, GREATER NEW YORK HOSPITAL ASSOCIATION

Ms. STREVEY. I have submitted a longer statement for the record, and I will try to summarize but using a little bit of the verbiage from the statement itself.

Good morning—no. Good afternoon. The statement says good morning. That is the first and hopefully only factual error.

Mr. TOWNS. I will take responsibility for that.

Ms. STREVEY. I am Elizabeth Sommers Strevey, the senior vice president for regulatory and professional affairs of the Greater New York Hospital Association.

Greater New York Hospital Association represents more than 155 not-for-profit and public hospitals and long-term care facilities in the five boroughs of New York and Westchester and Nassau County.

There are a significant number of emergency room visits in this country. In the United States, in 1991, more than 88 million emergency room visits took place. The hospitals that we represent served and provided 3 million of those 88 million visits. So we come to you as a representative of significant providers of emergency room services both in New York City and Nassau and Westchester Counties.

As has been reported, emergency departments in New York and other urban areas have been overwhelmed during the past several years by the sheer volume of patients seeking emergency department attention. While some point to the lack of an adequate primary care system for this, one must also take into account the societal ills which plague urban areas in particular when determining the root causes of increases in emergency department use.

The purpose of my particular statement today, because Dr. Primm is the real expert on substance abuse in the room, is to highlight issues relating to emergency room department crowding in the New York City area and to highlight, within that, the amount that may be related to substance abuse either directly or indirectly.

As you noted during Dr. Melnick's testimony, their study is a sampling of institutions and emergency departments.

Further I will try to outline a few positive steps that the Association and its members would find useful. In particular, Greater New York supports the efforts of the chairman to extend Federal Medicaid funding for residential substance treatment which would increase the availability of treatment and, consequently, help to alleviate emergency room backlogs related in part to substance abuse.

What have we been seeing? I point to the chart—I realize I did not number the page, but on the third page of the testimony we do have a small chart that we created in February of this year to highlight what is going on in the emergency rooms of New York City.

And as you will note, in the chairman's borough there were 79 available medical surgical beds in all of the hospitals in the Borough of Brooklyn.

On February 12, 1993, at that very same time and very same day, there were 208 patients waiting in emergency departments for beds and access to inpatient medical care. All of those patients are actually waiting in the emergency rooms in the five boroughs for access to a bed. And we believe some portion of that, perhaps more significant than we know, is related to substance abuse, either directly or indirectly.

There are 27,000 medical/surgical beds in the city of New York. So 727 available beds is as shown on the charts, a very small percentage of beds, in case you need to access those services.

Substance abuse in the emergency room: There is a fair amount of inpatient utilization and changes in terms of percentage of admissions related to substance abuse in comparison to other diagnoses. However, there are limited complete data—you can use the HHS study by extrapolation—to support the widely held belief that substance abuse cases have contributed markedly to emergency room overcrowding.

The chart on the fourth page of the testimony shows increases in the number of discharges related to substance abuse, patient days, and actual beds utilized by substance abuse patients.

Prior to this hearing, I questioned five emergency department directors of trauma centers because I wanted to get a handle, not only on the career substance abuse cases that we were seeing in our emergency departments but in the related cases, those that relate to trauma.

We have 15 trauma centers in New York City. We see more than 5,000 cases a year throughout that system. I asked each of five trauma center directors how much of the actual trauma they saw, in their professional opinion, was related to substance abuse. And by trauma, I meant gunshot wounds, stabbings, all of the things that relate to violence.

In each and every case, the emergency department directors of the five trauma centers were clear that while they had no statistics to justify their conclusion, they strongly suspected that more than 50 percent of the trauma cases they saw—some said as high as 90 percent and some as low as 50 percent—is related in some way to substance abuse; the seller, the buyer, the user, or the child or adult who got caught in between.

Therefore, while the data on inpatient admissions, those that enter with and are discharged with substance abuse diagnoses, show an increase. A more subtle, but more meaningful in terms of emergency room resource consumption, relationship can be drawn between substance abuse and visits to the ER because of trauma and trauma admissions.

I will agree with Congressman Rangel's statement that many of those, if we look back, would be difficult to find in the record because people don't have time when they are treating an acutely ill trauma patient to record all the dimensions of this problem.

There was a GAO study released in January that highlights issues of violence and illegal drugs in the emergency department utilization. We have included a couple of charts in the testimony from that report.

What can be done? There are no easy answers to the issue of overcrowded emergency departments. There are some actions that might facilitate solutions. One of the problems that continues to plague the health care system, patients, and providers alike, is the lack of adequate treatment options, particularly for those requiring methadone maintenance and residential drug treatment. And I note statistics about slots that are available and slots that are funded in the testimony.

I am sure some of you have heard of Beth Israel Medical Center in New York City which provides one of the largest networks of methadone maintenance clinics in the city. They have a waiting list of 300 patients, and those are patients who have cleared the academic and paperwork hurdles and are ready to go and seek treatment and get treatment at the time should it become available. That facility provided 58,000 emergency department visits between 1991 and 1992; and 5.3 percent were for problems directly related to substance abuse.

They also treated 8,000 patients in their methadone maintenance programs. And 14 percent of those patients required admission to the facility with half being admitted for substance abuse with half being admitted with medical diagnosis.

One of the issues that relates to the problems that precipitates itself on the emergency room is, without adequate treatment slots, patients also fall ill again for one reason or another. If discharge is delayed while we try to hunt for the appropriate treatment option—and not all options are appropriate for all patients—the patient may leave without an adequate discharge plan in place, because we cannot hold on to the patients. And patients often do not prefer our service to other things that may be available to them in the community. Without treatment, they run the higher risk of becoming HIV infected if they are not already, TB infected, if they are not already; and they may get discharged without seeking treatment at all.

If the hospital is not able to keep the patients, the patient leaves, continues to abuse substances, and continues to revisit the emergency department or even the inpatient setting.

Greater New York and its members, from their emergency departments' personnel to their discharge planners, would welcome additional assistance in providing for a more adequate number of treatment slots for those requiring post-acute care, outpatient, and residential services related to drug abuse.

Solving ED crowding will take many initiatives including rebuilding and expanding of the emergency departments. I know that you, Chairman Towns, have taken a lead in advocating for Federal Medicaid funding for residential substance abuse treatment, particularly for pregnant women and their family members.

We need funding to ensure financial viability emphasizing prevention and providing a mechanism to assure that people complete treatment.

Thank you.

Mr. TOWNS. Thank you.

[The prepared statement of Ms. Strevey follows:]

GNYHA
GREATER NEW YORK HOSPITAL ASSOCIATION
55 West 57th Street / New York, N.Y. 10019 / (212) 246-7100 / Fax (212) 262-6350
Kenneth E. Raske, President

TESTIMONY OF

ELIZABETH SOMMERS STREVEY

SENIOR VICE PRESIDENT

FOR REGULATORY AND PROFESSIONAL AFFAIRS

OF THE GREATER NEW YORK HOSPITAL ASSOCIATION

BEFORE THE

SUBCOMMITTEE ON HUMAN

RESOURCES AND INTERGOVERNMENTAL

RELATIONS OF THE GOVERNMENT OPERATIONS COMMITTEE

UNITED STATES HOUSE OF REPRESENTATIVES

ON

THE IMPACT OF INCREASED DRUG USE ON

EMERGENCY ROOM ADMISSION

WEDNESDAY, MAY 26, 1993

**TESTIMONY OF
ELIZABETH SOMMERS STREVEY
SENIOR VICE PRESIDENT
FOR REGULATORY AND PROFESSIONAL AFFAIRS
OF THE GREATER NEW YORK HOSPITAL ASSOCIATION
BEFORE THE
SUBCOMMITTEE ON HUMAN
RESOURCES AND INTERGOVERNMENTAL
RELATIONS OF THE GOVERNMENT OPERATIONS COMMITTEE
ON
THE IMPACT OF INCREASED DRUG USE ON
EMERGENCY ROOM ADMISSION
WEDNESDAY, MAY 26, 1993**

Good morning, Congressman Towns, members of the Subcommittee. I am Elizabeth Sommers Strevey, Senior Vice President for Regulatory and Professional Affairs of Greater New York Hospital Association (GNYHA). GNYHA represents the interests of 155 not-for-profit voluntary and public hospitals and long term care facilities in New York City and its surrounding communities. In the United States in 1991, according to the American Hospital Association, more than 88.5 million emergency room visits took place. I come before you today as a representative of those acute care institutions in our membership that, combined, provided more than 3,000,000 of those visits in their emergency departments to New York City residents and patients from elsewhere. GNYHA, therefore, represents institutions that are significant providers of emergency services in the New York City area and whose medical and administrative leaders are concerned about the rise in emergency department visits attributable either in part or in whole to substance abuse. According to the Health Systems Agency of New York City (HSA NYC), approximately 444,600 people in New York City can be classified as "heavy narcotic or non-narcotic abusers." Further, these people often seek health care through emergency rooms as many lack linkages to primary care services, according to a September, 1991, HSA NYC report.

As has been reported, emergency departments in New York City and other urban areas have been somewhat overwhelmed during the past several years by the sheer volume of patients seeking emergency department attention. While some may point to the lack of an adequate primary care system as the reason for this, one must also take into account the societal ills which plague urban areas in particular when determining the root causes of the increases in emergency department use.

The purpose of my statement today is to highlight issues related to emergency department crowding in the New York City area, in particular, during the past several years and to try to glean, within this scenario, the amount that may be related to substance abuse either directly or indirectly. Further, I will outline a few positive steps that may be taken in order to assist patients, facilities, and health care professionals in managing this issue. In particular, GNYHA supports the efforts of the Chairman to extend Federal Medicaid funding for residential substance abuse treatment which would increase the availability of treatment and, consequently, help to alleviate emergency room backlogs related in part to substance abuse.

THE CURRENT CONTEXT - Overcrowded Emergency Departments and New Epidemics

During the past several years, the emergency departments in the geographic area served by GNYHA, which is essentially the five boroughs of New York City, Nassau, and Westchester Counties, have experienced marked overcrowding, particularly in the winter months. At many times in New York City over the past several winters, there have been prolonged periods during which there were more patients awaiting admission to facilities than there were beds available. Additionally, the facilities that did manage to have some beds available during these particularly difficult times were not the facilities at which patients were awaiting admission. In some instances there were available beds at our specialty hospitals for orthopedics or eye and ear diseases. In other cases, where general service beds were open, patients have simply refused to be transferred or were too ill to be moved.

Below is a chart which shows how critically tight the situation was in emergency departments just as recently as February of this year. Data for years before would be similar. Given that New York City has approximately 27,000 acute care medical/surgical beds, these numbers are alarming.

Available Medical/Surgical Beds vs. Patients Awaiting Admission in the Emergency Room February 12, 1993

Borough	Available Medical/ Surgical Beds	Patients Awaiting Admission
Bronx	173	201
Brooklyn	79	208
Manhattan	369	187
Queens	86	143
Staten Island	20	31
New York City	727	770

While many have pointed to the twin epidemics of AIDS and tuberculosis as the reason for this additional strain on emergency departments, there are significant numbers of emergency department practitioners who would also point in another direction, namely substance abuse and related trauma.

There are no easy or obvious solutions to emergency department crowding. Even development of an adequate primary care network does not ensure that emergency departments will not continue to be extremely busy in the years ahead. However, the subject of this hearing today - substance abuse -- does play a role in the problem and can conceivably play a role in the solution.

SUBSTANCE ABUSE AND THE EMERGENCY DEPARTMENT - An Additional Set of Stresses and Strains

There is a fair amount of information on inpatient utilization and changes in terms of the percentage of admissions related to substance abuse in comparison to other diagnoses. However, there are limited data to support the widely held belief that substance abuse cases have contributed markedly to emergency department overcrowding. The chart below indicates the percentage change of discharges, patient days, and beds occupied due to substance abuse diagnoses as compared to psychiatric diagnoses for the past several years. If one is to assume that many of these patients, as is likely, entered the hospital through the emergency department, by extrapolation one can reasonably conclude that substance abuse contributes to emergency department crowding and increased emergency department utilization.

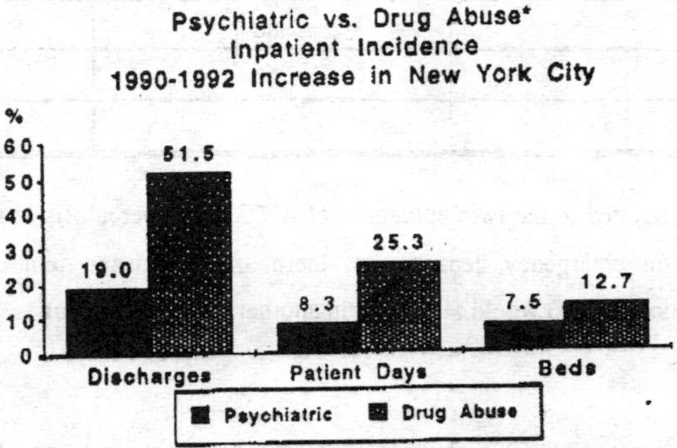

Source: United Hospital Fund
*Includes drug detoxification and rehabilitation

However, there are more subtle indications that, while not documented by GNYHA at this time, suggest that the significant rise in discharge diagnoses of substance abuse is only part of the equation. The recent U.S. Department of Health and Human Services study, which is referenced in the attached copy of an article which appeared in The New York Times, on April 24, 1993, confirms the perceptions of those on the frontlines.

Prior to this hearing, I questioned five emergency department directors of trauma centers in each of the five boroughs of New York City. I asked them, "How much of the actual trauma you see is, in your professional opinion, related to substance abuse?" By trauma I meant gunshot wounds, stabbings, etc. In each and every case, the emergency department directors of these five trauma centers were clear. While they had no statistics to justify their conclusion, they strongly suspected that more than 50% of the trauma cases they see (some said as much as 90%; some as low as 50%) is related in some way to substance abuse: the seller, the buyer, the user, or the person who got caught in between. Therefore, while the data on inpatient substance abuse admissions (those who enter with and essentially get discharged with a diagnosis of substance or drug abuse), show an increase, a more subtle (but meaningful in terms of emergency room resource consumption) relationship can be drawn between substance abuse and visits to the emergency room because of trauma and trauma admissions.

Further, data from the recently published U.S. Government Accounting Office (GAO) study on emergency departments confirms the significant presence of illegal drugs in already overburdened urban emergency departments.

Hospital EDs With Physician Examination Delays Have Other Contributing Factors
(Percent of Hospitals)

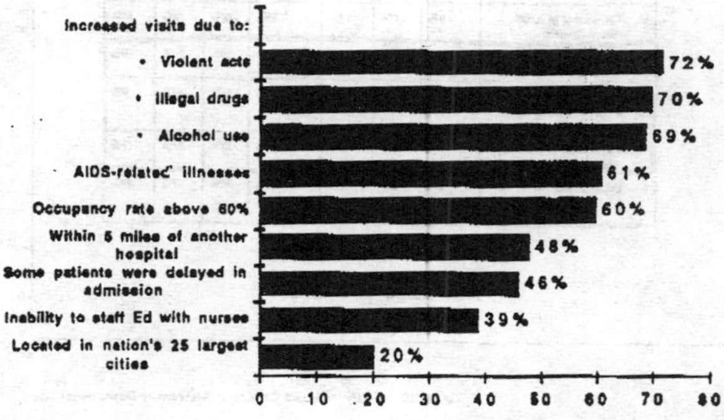

Source: U.S. General Accounting Office

The chart below, also from the GAO report, highlights and quantifies the perceptions of our local emergency department directors that substance abuse has increased, over time. Sixty-three percent of the responding emergency rooms, nationally, indicated that "the number of illegal drug-related medical problems" was on the increase.

17. Over the past 5 years, to what extent has each of the following increased, decreased or remained about the same in the geographic area served by your hospital? *(Check one box for each factor)*

(N=664-678, except (p.) N=30)	Decrease			Remained about the same	Increase		
	Significant	Moderate	Slight		Slight	Moderate	Significant
a. The incidence of illness	0%	1%	3%	46%	26%	24%	5%
b. The severity of illness	0%	<1%	1%	34%	22%	25%	17%
c. The number of people without health insurance	<1%	<1%	3%	14%	20%	30%	30%
d. The number of uninsured people seeking emergent health care	0%	<1%	1%	16%	24%	37%	22%
e. The number of insured people seeking emergent health care	2%	2%	8%	30%	37%	18%	6%
f. The number of people who are unemployed	0%	1%	3%	24%	34%	26%	12%
g. The number of people who are 65 years or older	0%	<1%	<1%	19%	33%	34%	14%
h. The number of primary care physicians	4%	7%	14%	38%	27%	11%	3%
i. The number of physicians who treat uninsured or publicly insured patients	9%	18%	22%	43%	5%	2%	1%
j. The number of public clinics that provide primary care	4%	7%	7%	70%	9%	3%	<1%
k. The number of people who do not have a regular physician	1%	1%	3%	31%	31%	25%	8%
l. The number of AIDS-related illnesses	0%	0%	<1%	12%	42%	25%	17%
m. The number of alcohol-related illnesses or injuries	0%	1%	3%	32%	33%	24%	8%
n. The number of illegal drug-related medical problems	<1%	<1%	3%	34%	34%	20%	9%
o. The number of violence-related injuries	0%	0%	1%	35%	32%	21%	11%
p. Other *(Specify)*	3%	0%	0%	10%	16%	30%	30%

Hospital Emergency Departments, 1991

GAO/HRD-93-4 Growth and Change in Emergency Department Use

WHAT CAN BE DONE?

While there are no easy answers to the issues of overcrowded emergency departments and to the related substance abuse issues, there are some actions that might facilitate solutions. One of the problems that continues to plague the health care system - its patients and its providers alike - is the lack of an adequate supply of treatment options for substance abusing patients, particularly those requiring methadone maintenance and residential drug treatment. According to the Bureau of Program Reporting of the New York State Office of Alcoholism and Substance Abuse Services (OASAS), the total treatment capacity in New York City is 53,000 slots, of which OASAS funds 37,000 slots.

At one of the institutions in New York City that itself controls the largest network of methadone maintenance programs, Beth Israel Medical Center, the waiting list for all of its programs is approximately 300 people seeking treatment. There are many others who would clearly benefit, but they are not willing to pursue the process. This institution provides inpatient detoxification and substance abuse services, a full service emergency department, and an extraordinary number of outpatient treatment options for patients with substance abuse problems. However, even this institution, with such a comprehensive array of services cannot meet the demands that its own patients place on it for substance abuse treatment. This facility provided 58,009 visits in its emergency department between December, 1991, and November, 1992. Of these visits, 3,094 (or 5.3%) were for problems directly related to substance abuse or alcohol abuse. No accounting was available on the trauma-related visits.

This hospital also treated 8,000 patients in its many methadone maintenance programs between 1989 and 1990. Of the 8,000 patients, approximately 14% required admission to the facility with half of the 14% being admitted for problems related to drug detoxification. This case study exemplifies the larger system's issues.

Patients who must be discharged from the hospital because they are no longer acutely ill must have adequate discharge plans arranged. However, the hospital cannot retain a patient who simply wishes to leave. If discharge is delayed because treatment options are unavailable and waiting times for discharge are extended, problems may occur:

- The patient leaves without an adequate discharge plan in place and waits, without treatment, for an available slot in a drug treatment program. Sometimes, patients get discouraged about seeking treatment at all.
- If the hospital is not able to keep the patient, the patient leaves, continues to abuse substances and revisits the emergency department or even the inpatient setting.

GNYHA and its members -- from their emergency departments' personnel and their inpatient substance abuse detoxification service personnel to their discharge planners – would welcome additional assistance in providing for a more adequate number of treatment slots for those requiring post acute care outpatient and residential services related to drug abuse. Solving the emergency department crowding will take many initiatives including rebuilding and expanding emergency departments. To get at the root causes of the problem will require providing an adequate number of treatment options, securing funding for their financial viability, emphasizing prevention, and providing a mechanism to assure that persons complete treatment.

I know that you, Chairman Towns, have taken the lead in advocating for Federal Medicaid funding for residential substance abuse treatment, particularly for pregnant women and their family members. As you know, the Federal Medicaid program prohibits reimbursement for services provided in "institutions for mental diseases," or "IMDs," for Medicaid-eligible individuals aged 22 to 64. Because the Health Care Financing Administration has classified substance abuse as a mental illness, residential substance abuse treatment facilities have been classified as IMDs and have been denied Medicaid reimbursement. The promise of a stable reimbursement stream through the Federal Medicaid program, as you have called for, could go a long way toward ensuring the development of the additional substance abuse treatment slots which are critically needed to alleviate emergency room overcrowding.

We thank you for the opportunity to testify here today on this subject of critical importance to the well being of the citizens of New York and the health care providers.

Emergency Hospital Visits Rise Among Drug Abusers

By JOSEPH B. TREASTER

Though casual drug use in America has been dropping, the latest Government statistics on emergency-room visits show that problems among the heaviest users have risen to record levels.

The emergency-room statistics released yesterday show that drugs are taking an increasing toll on poor inner-city neighborhoods whose hospital emergency rooms are already stretched to the limit. They also show that heroin is causing an increasing proportion of the health problems that bring people to the hospital.

"Serious drug problems persist in our country," said Donna E. Shalala, the Secretary of Health and Human Services, adding that the problems "affect individuals, undermine communities and impact heavily on our health-care system."

Rise Is After Decline

The increase in emergency-room visits is particularly striking because it comes after several years in which overall drug use dropped drastically. According to the latest Government surveys on drug consumption, 1.9 million Americans used cocaine in 1991, compared with 5.8 million in 1985.

But the hospital statistics made public yesterday by the Substance Abuse and Mental Health Services Administration in Dr. Shalala's department showed that 30,924 people sought emergency-room help from July to September 1992 because of cocaine abuse, compared with 28,552 people a year earlier, an increase of 8.2 percent.

Sharpest Rise in Heroin Cases

And the rise in heroin-related problems was even steeper. Last summer, 13,387 people sought emergency-room help because of problems with heroin, compared with 10,338 for the same period a year earlier, an increase of nearly 30 percent.

The previous records were reached in the summer of 1989, when 12,095 people sought emergency-room help because of heroin abuse and 29,939 because of cocaine. Drug-induced emergency-room visits then fell sharply, and stayed down for more than a year before starting to rise again in early 1991.

Drug experts in law enforcement and treatment said that while the latest hospital statistics were collected nearly a year ago, there is no sign of a shift in the trend. "We've seen nothing to indicate a decline," said Dr. Mitchell S. Rosenthal, the president of Phoenix House, one of the nation's largest residential drug-treatment organizations.

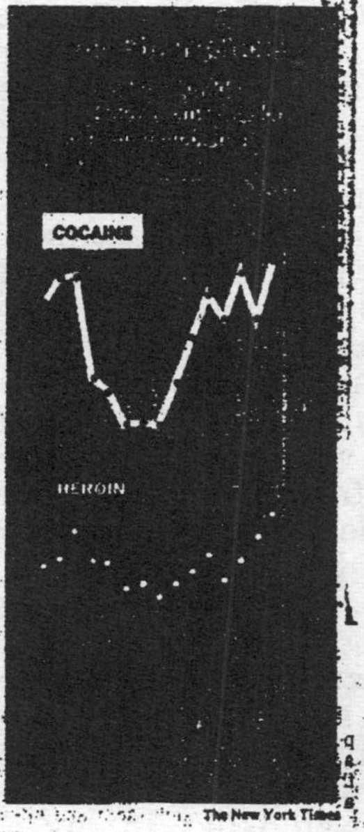

The New York Times

Robert A. Bryden, the head of the Drug Enforcement Administration office in New York, said heroin trafficking is increasing in the city and that cocaine trafficking has remained constant at a high level.

"There is increased production of drugs overseas and increased smuggling," he said, "and there is an increased appetite among drug users in New York. I think this is typical of most of the big cities."

The Clinton Administration has made little progress toward developing a drug policy. The nation's top drug-fighting job, the White House Office of National Drug Control Policy, is empty, as are other important Government drug positions. And President Clinton's new budget has been criticized by drug experts for continuing the emphasis of previous Administrations on law enforcement, to the detriment of rehabilitation and education.

Mr. Bryden said the rise in emergency-room visits because of heroin abuse show the need for better education, particularly as young users are beginning to sniff and smoke heroin. "Every kid in school knows that injecting heroin is bad for you," he said, "but I'm just not sure we've done enough to get out the word that smoking and sniffing is highly addictive and just as dangerous."

Treatment Spending May Rise

White House officials say that the overhaul of the national health-care system being studied by the task force, headed by Hillary Rodham Clinton, is likely to include increases in spending on drug treatment. But they have provided no details.

"While this problem did not occur on President Clinton's watch, it is now his problem," said Dr. Herbert D. Kleber, an executive of the Center on Addiction and Substance Abuse at Columbia University and a former official in the Bush Administration. "It will not go away if ignored."

Treating people with drug problems in emergency rooms is much more expensive than programs intended to wean them away from drugs, said Dr. Kleber. Moreover, he said, heavy drug users have a high rate of infection with the virus that causes AIDS, and they have played a leading role in the nation's tuberculosis epidemic.

Mr. Rosenthal of Phoenix House, who also heads Gov. Mario M. Cuomo's council on substance abuse, said he has been struck by what he describes as President Clinton's lack of attention to the drug problem.

"The stunning paradox," he said, "is that we have a President who says he is focusing on health care and on the domestic agenda. And here we have something that is causing health problems, impacting on child welfare, housing, education, so many things, and we're not talking about it."

Mr. TOWNS. And Dr. Primm.

STATEMENT OF BENY J. PRIMM, EXECUTIVE DIRECTOR, ADDICTION RESEARCH AND TREATMENT CORP., BROOKLYN, NY

Dr. PRIMM. Thank you, Mr. Towns.

Mr. Chairman, I first want to congratulate you for calling the hearing. And certainly I want to thank the members of the committee, Mr. Washington and Mr. Payne, and certainly you too, where I have programs in your district and these gentlemen have been of considerable help to me since I have been in Washington, and I am extremely grateful for that.

The 24th of this month was my last day as a consultant to the agency that I serve in, the Center for Substance Abuse Treatment, at SAMHSA. My last official day as director of that office was, of course, February 24; and I spent the last 3 months as a consultant to the acting—and I want to emphasize that—the acting director of the Center for Substance Abuse Treatment.

The reason I preface whatever I have to say with that remark is because, today I am free of the bond and the bondage that has certainly not allowed me to say a number of things that I would have liked to have said because of possible problems or repercussions that it would create.

And today I can be open and more forthcoming that I ever have because I am now a citizen, Beny J. Primm, who is the director of the Addiction Research and Treatment Corp. that you know, Mr. Chairman, and the Urban Institute that serves both Harlem, Brooklyn, Queens and the great State of New York.

So with that over, I would like to say a couple of things first about the DAWN report, which it is one of the few things that we have in terms of data collection out there that can give us some ideas.

As a matter of fact, you called this hearing based on the fact that you possibly were shocked at some of the things that you saw in the DAWN report. So at least it serves some good there.

But I wish that I could be so specialized as Dr. Melnick stated that he is and as he picks up what is happening with the DAWN data being collected in hospitals that he can only focus on how the impact of this is on hospital emergency rooms secondary to the use of drugs or illicit drugs and some, of course, licit drugs.

Let me say that I think those numbers would be much, much higher if they were related to tuberculosis that we are seeing in these populations. Certainly, HIV infection or AIDS and the related problems that AIDS have caused and the plethora of problems that are created by addictive behavior, subacute bacterial endocarditis, Hepatitis A and B and all of these diseases that are plaguing the population that we are trying to target and serve.

I would also like for the specialty of data collection or DAWN to focus more on who are these people who come. Not their names or their number. We don't need to know their names. We know that most of them are black because we saw here that a number of these individuals who came, there was an increase in 35-years olds and an increase in blacks using heroin and cocaine. And I can talk about that, because from that data—certainly I go out and visit programs and my own program in New York and talk to people who work in hospital emergency rooms. And I have a damn good notion why 35-year-old black men and 35-year-old men who are out there living in this socioeconomic climate are now using more heroin and using more cocaine.

I think Congressman Rangel made it very clear that certainly that is the problem. I also have a notion why it is reported in the press that 35 years old and younger men in our country are becoming more depressed we have almost caught up with women in terms of depression. It is because of the socioeconomic climate. There is no question about it. If we related some of these visits to the other problems that are occurring in society we could extrapolate from that knowledge and focus on the problems in our Nation that affects particular individuals.

I also think that in Dr. Melnick's office, in SAMHSA, has 35 people. I don't know how much we paid for the DAWN program. I have no idea. It is in the millions of dollars. I think that such a number of personnel and the amount of money that we pay could give us far more than we get from that particular survey and others that are done.

And I mean, when you have 35 people, which is far more than the Office of National Drug Control Policy—they only have 25—that is what has been recommended, and that is what the President says at the executive branch they will have—you can do more than just focus on the impact that it has on the emergency rooms.

You may recall, Mr. Chairman, when you were at Harlem Hospital that I was a young anesthesiologist at that time with no gray hair and certainly——

Mr. TOWNS. I didn't have any either.

Dr. PRIMM. That is right. You may recall that I set up what was called the hospital orientation center. This was some-30 years ago today. And in that center what we did is exactly what she reported on today, and that is that we focused in emergency rooms on the number of people that came in and had either a direct relationship to narcotic addiction or an indirect relationship and we counted during that time 30 years ago at Harlem Hospital Center that 85 percent of all the surgical cases done on an emergency basis were either directly or indirectly related to narcotic addiction. That is the kind of data that we need to see.

We also need to see when we collect data like the DAWN data, who are these people that come into the emergency room? Are they employed? Why are they in the emergency room? When you go into an emergency room, for example, it is very interesting that you have to wait 4 to 5 or 6 hours to be helped.

It is humiliating and dehumanizing in many instances. There are other people in the emergency room, all poor people, many of them. And we know that tuberculosis is a disease of poverty, and we are associating HIV with that problem. So those people that come to that place have no access, generally to other kinds of medical care that would be commensurate with the kind of care that you and I got. So we need to know more from those kinds of studies.

I would also like to talk for just a moment, Mr. Chairman, about comprehensiveness. You heard this morning Mr. Rangel talk about comprehensiveness. He talked about the approach to the problem should be a comprehensive approach, one that not only targets just the host, the individual, but the chemical itself in terms of interdiction both at the community level and at the national and international levels, but also the environment in which that individual lives. And hardly anybody has said anything about that situation. If we don't correct that environment and don't do it on a very national scale, we are not going to make an impact on this problem.

What do I mean by that? I would like to cite during my own tenure here that I began to link agencies as much as I could so that they could focus on the problem in a comprehensive manner. We are talking about the Department of Labor, the Department of Education, the Department of Housing and Urban Development, along with HHS, and the Department of Education, all doing their job.

And we need to target those critical populations, which this particular problem sorely affects. And we haven't done that. If we are talking about a partnership for a drug-free America, we are targeting the American population. That is great. There is nothing wrong with that. I think we should compliment the media, TV, the print media, and whatever.

But on the other hand, it was not targeted at the problem where it is the greatest in the inner city where you and I come from, and targeting it is not culturally distinct nor is it in a manner where people could embrace it and begin to do something about it.

Certainly we saw reduction in substance abuse in certain populations, but we have seen a rise in heroin and cocaine abuse in other populations. And I think that is important that we target the educational message toward them and we have not done so, nor have we spent adequately enough.

I think the whole problem—someone mentioned smoking, one of the Congress persons who was here this morning earlier and its impact—let me give you an example what happened at the Substance Abuse and Mental Health Services Administration when I tried to include in my announcements that anybody receiving a discretionary grant from the Center for Substance Abuse Treatment in the Nation, any provider, that they should have a nonsmoking policy because this is a health problem. OK?

And substance abuse is a health problem. And if we are going to fund people to do something about rehabilitation of addicts certainly in the edifice where this takes place there should not be another deleterious substance that could cause other problems and exacerbate the health problems that are there. I had to fight in order to get even such a soft statement in my announcement. I think that kind of thing, that kind of bureaucratic control over clinicians who are brought to Washington to make things better for the people that you all represent makes it very difficult for us to get our job done.

I would like, also, Mr. Chairman, in closing my opening statement, to talk about some of the things that I think that I have recognized since I have been here that are a little bit of a problem. The Federal Government in Health and Human Services and the newly created SAMHSA in October 1992, I thought was set up to specifically focus on substance abuse and mental health problems and to help that provider constituency and the consumer constituency that we target out there.

It is very difficult for us to do so. It is difficult because of the bureaucratic layers that are involved therein in the system. It is difficult for us to hire minority candidates or search out minority candidates because the hiring process is a problem, which means that many of the policies that are set up have no input from those individuals who are going to be affected by those policies.

And I think that is something that Congress should look into and pay very close attention to it. Now, as a private citizen, I certainly am going to be in contact with you, Mr. Chairman, and other Members of Congress to try to let you know what is going on, because I don't think Congress is all that well versed about what goes on in these departments that so sorely affect individuals of color in this Nation and our communities.

With that, Mr. Chairman, I would like to close my formal opening and say, sir, I would love to respond to any questions that you might have surrounding this issue.

Mr. TOWNS. Let me thank both of you, Dr. Strevey and Dr. Primm, for your testimony.

Dr. Primm, let me start with you. Let me open by saying that I admire the kind of work that you have done over the years in New York. Over the past 30 years, I think you were in the forefront of recognizing that there was a problem and moving to try to deal with the problem. And so I want to first applaud you for that.

Dr. PRIMM. Thank you.

Mr. TOWNS. But I also want to look very carefully at your past 4 years here. You have spent the last approximately 4 years establishing the Office of Treatment Improvement, now the Center of Substance Abuse Treatment.

Would you share with this committee what you see as your successes? What worked best in the center? And in those areas that were not too successful, what would it have taken to have made them successful?

In the opening, you said that you are no longer a part of it so you can speak freely, so I want to take the opportunity to give you a chance to do that, because we want to learn from you. I think you are one person in this country that we all can learn from. You have had experience in almost every area of work.

Dr. PRIMM. If I could begin to highlight some of the things that I think the office accomplished under my leadership, was certainly the recruitment of dedicated and culturally diverse staff that were committed to improving the delivery of services for treatment of substance abuse.

We started out with 14 people. I wanted you to hear that; 14 people on my staff in late 1989, 1990. The office was established January 1, 1990. And let me tell you, for the next 9 months we managed a budget, and we grew to 27 people and $1.336 billion with not enough direct operating funds because we were created as an office of the Office of the Administrator and as a consequence had very little money to do the job.

Now we have grown to 160 people and are more able to do the job. And I cite that because when we talk about the establishment of a new office with a mission to improve drug treatment in our

Nation, Congress has to see to it and be a watchdog over that agency to make sure that they give that individual who they bring here enough money and enough staff to carry out the mission of that office.

We also developed what I think was some excellent pieces of literature that went out to the States, treatment improvement protocol statements and treatment improvement exchange statements where we tell the States—give them a "how to," just recommendations; we don't tell them they must do this but recommendations of how to do things.

We established a variety of treatment complexes in our Nation that linked the human immunodeficiency virus, tuberculosis, and other diseases that plague this population so that it doesn't go on to branch out into the other communities and have made the Nation pretty much aware, particularly in the treatment field about these issues.

We structured and implemented what is, I feel, for pregnant and postpartum women and infants who were exposed to drugs and—I heard a person refer to crack babies. In California 80,000 will be born this year. I think we need to get rid of that term, Mr. Chairman, and talk about babies exposed to drugs, because that crack baby designation follows that child throughout their career and maybe we expect negative consequences from that child.

I have had the opportunity, of course, to work with some very dedicated people in Congress that have helped create comprehensive approaches to substance abuse treatment. I think we have expanded drug treatment capacity, and we have improved drug treatment. I would have liked to have had a greater flexibility, Mr. Chairman, in managing substance abuse treatment. I found that there were a lot of inertia in the bureaucratic set up here in Washington which I think could be looked at a little bit more closely so people could better do their job.

I only hope that the leadership that I put in place at the Center for Substance Abuse Treatment will be able to carry on some of these comprehensive ideas. And with Congress sort of watch dogging, I think it can happen.

And that, in brevity, is what we have done. I can certainly submit in writing to you other things that I feel would expand on this to give you a better understanding.

I have had contact, of course, with Mr. Washington and Mr. Payne and Mr. Rangel and so forth, Mr. Stockings. I visited their cities and made sure that areas that needed the focus, got the focus. And I am in constant communication with Congress, and I hope to still be in that same relationship.

Mr. TOWNS. I want you to know that was not any intention to be a loaded question, because I have great admiration and respect for you. And I think that the bright spot over there was you.

I think you were one of the members of that staff that we all respected here on this side of the town. And I wanted to share that with you. I just wish this administration would recognize that and find a way to bring you back in because if they are serious about combating the problem, then we need the best minds and the people with experience.

I say that for the record, though you sort of made up your mind. But the point is that I hope that somewhere along the line they will look and see the kind of service that you provided in our war on drugs. I think that having a war on drugs without having you as a part of a fight will not work. I don't know how much we are doing.

Let me yield to Congressman Washington and ask him to take the Chair, please.

Mr. WASHINGTON [presiding]. Thank you, Mr. Chairman.

Since I am in the Chair, I will yield to Mr. Horn.

Mr. HORN. Thank you, Mr. Chairman.

Dr. Primm, since you mentioned that perhaps the term "crack babies" was inappropriate and we ought to talk about those——

Dr. PRIMM. The term. The term.

Mr. HORN. The term—and we ought to talk about the babies addicted to drugs——

Dr. PRIMM. Exposed to drugs.

Mr. HORN. Exposed—what is the best scientific thinking as to what will happen to these babies should they survive their first years? And what are the likely predictions, because of the drugs that they were exposed to through the ignorance of their mothers, usually, and what kind of behavior will that lead to and what kind of problem does that pose for the school system and the society in general?

Dr. PRIMM. The jury is still out on infants exposed to sedative hypnotics and stimulants. We know that some early signs, delayed development, delayed learning, specifically feeding problems early on, developmental problems early on, which all could possibly lead to some developmentally disabled problems later on in life.

But we have not yet, I don't feel, done enough study to say that these kids are going to be any more burdensome later on in life if they are put into the right kinds of programs as they develop. Unquestionably, it is a different impact. Drugs have a different impact on the developmental state and evolution of these children than on other individuals who are not exposed to drugs.

But we are also looking at cigarettes and also at alcohol. The fetal alcohol syndrome poses the same problem. And probably alcohol has a greater impact on these individuals than indeed does cocaine and other stimulant drugs.

Mr. HORN. Do we have any longitudinal studies underway to make these comparisons to track these poor little children for the next 5 to 10 to 20 years.

Dr. PRIMM. There are a number of studies sponsored by the National Institute on Drug Abuse and by the office that I just left, for treatment, not for research.

There is research being done by the National Institute on Drug Research. And we are following them and their mothers both for in-house treatment and also for outpatient treatment of these individuals with their mothers with them.

So, yes, there are studies going on.

Mr. HORN. How long has this phenomenon been going on? When did it first become noticeable?

Dr. PRIMM. Probably around 1983 to 1984 we began to see, in New York, a rise in the use of crack cocaine and an increase in sexually transmitted diseases and an increased number of babies being born positive for syphilis and certainly affected by cocaine.

Great numbers of people began to practice different sexual behaviors and to prostitute themselves to get cocaine and were exposed to all these different problems.

So that is when we began to really notice it, about 1983. But the trend probably started in 1981, and it has gone up gradually ever since that time. And there has been followup ever since that time also.

Mr. HORN. What would you suggest in educating the mothers involved? And what is New York doing in this area?

Dr. PRIMM. I think we need to target the areas where we see an increase or a hotbed of this kind of problem. We have not done so.

Sometimes we have not done so because community leaders may say that the African American community or the Hispanic community already has enough burden to bear, let alone putting this particular problem on their community.

I speak out very strongly both in African American communities and to my white colleagues who happen to be in positions to recognize some of the data and interpret some of the data that indicates where these problems are and tell them, we would much better be considered racists in our views now than a conspirator down the line 10 years from now when the problem really hits.

And I have encouraged them that no matter what the burden is, that if it is a health care problem—and the data shows this, we are seeing 35-year-old men, for example, increase in drug use, both heroin and cocaine use. We are seeing black men, 35 years and older—we have to target that and make that public. No matter whether it hurts or not because health statistics or data tells us that, and we better do something about it or it is going to get worse and not just say we are seeing younger people not involved and so this thing is going to go down when they reach 35 or in a few years from now.

I think we should look at these trends and data and extrapolate from them what we need and go out there and do the job rather than to say, well, it is just an impact on the emergency room. I see a broadening—I wish I could be so specialized and not see the housing, the unemployed, the wall-to-wall people on the street corners who are standing there either drinking or drugging. OK?

I know what that means, and I know what that comes from. That nucleus of people spreads out, and my whole community deteriorates. The whole economy of the community is eroded by that kind of behavior. People buy each other's television sets and my radio from my Mercedes, et cetera.

I need not tell you, Mr. Horn, how important some of these things are to me. The fire burns in my belly as it did 35 years ago as a young anesthesiologist. I made twice as much money then as I ever have done since, and I dedicated myself to this problem because I think it is the most neglected, untargeted group of people in our Nation. And it will remain to plague us ad infinitum.

Mr. HORN. Over the years, public schools have had courses for health. What is your opinion of how much help, if any, these courses in the public schools can deal with this public problem?

Can we educate 14 to 17-year old females in particular who are likely to get pregnant, you know, getting pregnant and perhaps being a mother?

Is any progress being made in that area?

Dr. PRIMM. I think so. I think a number of social organizations in our Nation who were set up primarily as social organizations have begun to focus on that. And I can give you an example of some of them.

Some of the African American sororities and African American women's organization have set up programs where they actually go into a communities and target young women just like you are talking about. Unquestionably.

I think this has been raised because we are seeing the result of these problems particularly in minority communities. And people of serious import, both in the social setting, the political setting, and unquestionably in the educational setting, have begun to do something about it. There is utilization of the schools now in those hours when schools are closed.

I often wondered why shouldn't churches and schools be used for that purpose? I and the Office of Substance Abuse Treatment began a whole focus on the religious community with clergy, teaching them about a community ministry where they themselves begin to target people and to recreate the extended family like I once had as I grew up.

In my neighborhood, when I grew up, if I did something wrong, I may have gotten a beaten by somebody 2 or 3 times before I got home. And then I got another one when I got home. That doesn't exist anymore. Teachers can no longer monitor and discipline the children the way they once did.

That is being recreated in communities. People are taking over their communities. They no longer want advertisements in their communities for the children, like what is happening in Harlem and in Baltimore and Atlanta, GA, where the young people have organized to do something about the advertisements; 100,000 kids will have seen 100,000 advertisements for cigarettes and liquor by the time they are 16 years old. That is incredible and hypocritical.

We have, on the front cover of one of our magazines: "Drug Abuse and Crack, Do Something About It." And on the back of the magazine we have, "Old Grand Dad." We shouldn't allow Time magazine to have such a hypocritical approach to the problem. I have slides that depict Mayor Barry on the front page of Newsweek and on the back, advertising liquor on the back page. It is ridiculous. You see my point?

I think, yes, the Congress needs to focus on it. We need to focus on it. Clergy needs to focus on it. And we are seeing that in certain communities.

Mr. HORN. Thank you. I appreciate the testimony of both of you.

Dr. PRIMM. Thank you, Mr. Horn.

Mr. WASHINGTON. I would like to ask a question of both of you. What is the methodology by which scientists quantify proportionately between various kinds of drugs to determine which is most addictive?

Dr. PRIMM. Well, there are animal experiments, and I know that is a real buzz word when you begin to talk about that. My former boss was pretty much put out of his job because he talked about experiments that compared monkeys with humans and particular humans that live in the inner city. So I don't want to be misstated on this fact.

But the only way we know about drugs and the extent or the degree of their addictive potential is to look at them initially in animals. And we know that the most addictive of all drugs—and this may shock you—and that is amphetamines.

Probably the second most addictive is cocaine because of what it does to the higher centers.

Because of what we have seen, if you place cocaine or amphetamines in a vial mixed with a solution and hook that up to a chimpanzee or a rhesus monkey, that they will continue to press the lever to get this shot until they die, disregarding sex, disregarding food, and every other vital thing for them; they will take the cocaine as a choice. If there is cocaine and amphetamines, they will take the amphetamines as a choice. We know that.

We also know that heroin and other opiate derivatives, too, are addictive, not necessarily as addictive as are other stimulants that I just mentioned.

Mr. WASHINGTON. So the comparison is a gross comparison? And we are unable to quantify it?

Dr. PRIMM. Quantify it? You mean the amount of a drug——

Mr. WASHINGTON. No. I mean you couldn't say—it sounds partly theoretical, if I may. And I can understand the example you gave where you use an animal or a monkey and you give her or him choices and based upon their choices, you reach certain theoretical conclusions as to which one they like the most and thereby deduce that the one they like the most is the one that is the most addictive.

That is basically what you said, isn't it?

Dr. PRIMM. Yes.

Mr. WASHINGTON. But you couldn't say one is 37 percent addictive and one is 14 percent addictive.

Dr. PRIMM. Well, if you put it on a scale like that, we know that the use of crack cocaine, that is if you inhale it like crack cocaine, you smoke it, it is far more addictive and creates addiction far quicker because it gets to the brain within 6 to 7 seconds when you smoke it.

Mr. WASHINGTON. That is because of the method of inducement and not the properties of the drug.

Dr. PRIMM. The physical properties of the drug play a significant role in its effect. It is introduced as a gas and goes directly to the brain in a very short period of time, even somewhat faster than intravenous cocaine would go.

Mr. WASHINGTON. Do we know how much more addictive crack cocaine is in comparison with powdered cocaine?

Dr. PRIMM. Well, I think there are some studies. I wish I could cite a particular study for you. The pharmacodynamics of the two forms of the drug are similar, depending upon which way they are taken.

If you insufflate, if you snort it, for example, the onset is longer than if you smoke it or take it subcutaneously.

Mr. WASHINGTON. You are going into a mucous membrane and into the blood that way.

Dr. PRIMM. And it is absorbed rather fast because one of the most vascularized areas of the body is, of course, the nose, the mucous membrane of the nose.

I wish I could, on a scale of 0 to 100, say cocaine is 100 percent addictive and crack cocaine is 102 or whatever and then below that, marijuana, you become dependent, but you may not become addicted, et cetera.

There are scales like that. Off the top of my head, I don't—I could submit something for the record and cite the literature.

Mr. WASHINGTON. Mine is a general concern. My attention was called to a story on the front page of USA Today in today's paper in which a comparison was made as between powdered cocaine and crack cocaine, based upon information from the U.S. Sentencing Commission, it is drug of choice of most African American males, crack cocaine.

Those figures were more evenly divided between Hispanic males, African American males and Anglo males with respect to powdered cocaine. And across the board, in general, the punishment is about 5 times more severe for crack cocaine.

And I just wanted to know whether the addictive effects was 5 times greater which would then make the punishment fit the crime. And if not, I am troubled by that.

Dr. PRIMM. You should be troubled Mr. Washington. Both are addictive. One may act faster than the other in terms of getting to the brain and causing its impact, but, unquestionably, that is a matter of seconds rather than a matter of whatever. But the severity of addiction is the same.

I would say that our criminal justice system certainly does target certain behaviors among certain people and treat them more draconian than they do the same behavior among other people. We know that about 68 percent of all the drug abuse in this Nation is by white people. It is a fact, OK?

And we know that if we look at the number of people who are in jail, secondary to drug problems, we are talking 50 to 60 percent are black people or Hispanic people. That is very interesting.

It has been explained by people in the criminal justice system that a lot of minorities are low-level dealers and, therefore, you see them more and they are arrested more. I think we are more targeted, to be frank with you. When I drive my Mercedes with a top down, and I am a physician in this country with 40 years, I am very afraid that I am going to be stopped. And I have been. I have been. I can show you that I have been stopped because I was dressed dirty that day washing my car and working on my yard and they said I am just checking you. Can I see your license and registration. And I said, for what? And he said I am just checking you. And I said I am going home. You follow me home that is where my license and registration are. And if you want to arrest me, you can.

We are targeted. And just because you are a Congressman, you have that bow tie and nice suit and you sit here today does not mean that when you go out in the street that you are not targeted as a black man in this country.

Mr. WASHINGTON. I have known for a long time that I am not free. I am just loose.

Dr. PRIMM. I might have said this morning that my bonds were off of me. But I know that I, too, am not free. And I said today, and I felt comfortable in doing so, Mr. Washington, to say exactly what I have seen and felt because I think Congress must know.

You are, to me, the last bastion of help as a pop-off valve for the provider and the consumer of the services that you want us to render to this Nation. It is not at HHS. It is not the Secretary. It is not the administrator of SAMHSA. It is Congress.

And that is why I was so happy when notified to come here today to testify and to do anything else that you may like.

Mr. WASHINGTON. Thank you, both you, very much for your testimony. You have added a great deal to the body of knowledge that will be before the Congress. And I assure you that not only the testimony you give today but the spirit in which you give it will be embodied as we continue our work to try to deal with this most pressing and most important issue that faces our Nation.

And as you both indicated in your testimony, we are, perhaps, only looking at the tip of the iceberg—and it seems to me that we have to be serious about what we do and must take the benefit and counsel of all three of you, and of course of Congressman Rangel who is not here, and interweave it, if you will, into the work that we do, because it ought to be apparent to us that we can't continue to throw money at the problem and expect results; we can't anoint something and call it a war and thereby ensure that we will be successful.

We can't even have a military siege type mentality in dealing with the problem. We must be more responsible and responsive in the way in which we treat what is a public health problem in our country.

And I assure you that the work that you do does not go unnoticed, and the testimony you have given will be taken into serious consideration.

And on behalf of the chairman and all of the members of the committee, I would like to thank you for your testimony.

The hearing stands adjourned.

Dr. PRIMM. Thank you, Congressman. Thank you very much.

[Whereupon, at 12:52 p.m., the subcommittee adjourned, to reconvene subject to the call of the Chair.]

○

85-837 (96)